I0094360

the
MODERN
PARENT

Raising a great kid in
the digital world

MARTINE OGLETHORPE

Copyright © 2020 Martine Oglethorpe

All rights reserved. No part of this book may be reproduced by any mechanical, photographic, or electronic process, or in the form of a phonographic recording, nor may it be stored in a retrieval system, transmitted, or otherwise be copied for public or private use—other than for 'fair use' as brief quotations embodied in articles and reviews—without prior written permission of the publisher.

The information in this book is true and complete to the best of the author's knowledge. Any advice or recommendations are made without guarantee on the part of the author or publisher. The author and publisher disclaim any liability in connection with the use of this information.

Published in Australia by The Modern Parent

Printed in Australia

First Edition

National Library of Australia Cataloguing-in-Publication entry available for this title at nla.gov.au

ISBN: 978-0-6488286-0-0

Cover and Interior Design: Swish Design

Front and Back Cover Images: Janis House Photography

For Oliver, Charlie, Will, Ava, Louie and Alfie

CONTENTS

the
MODERN PARENT

MARTINE OGLETHORPE

FOREWORD

Michael Grose—Founder, Parenting Ideas

Digital technology has changed the parenting territory dramatically in recent years. I've seen nothing in my 30 years as a parenting educator that has fundamentally changed the parenting landscape like the emergence of digital technology. Suddenly we've been tasked with preparing kids to be safe, happy and successful, not just in the real world, but in the online world as well. This is new territory for most parents as no matter how tech-savvy you are, there was probably little in your family of origin that prepared you for the challenges you now face.

Martine Oglethorpe is part of the new breed of parenting educator who nimbly stays abreast of technology changes, yet keeps one foot firmly grounded in the timeless ways that make families strong. I came across Martine's work some time ago and loved her positive, no-nonsense approach to raising kids in this new digital and social media space. Suddenly there was someone opening up possibilities and helping us peer into the opportunities that digital technology offers our kids—but always with our eyes wide open.

This book is the very best of Martine Oglethorpe. It takes the fear out of parenting kids in the digital age and replaces it with confidence and optimism. Martine skilfully combines her professional expertise with her experiences of guiding her own children down the pathway to being skilled, savvy digital citizens. In these pages lies the blueprint for parenting kids in the digital age; that is, to be engaged in children's digital lives without being overbearing or burdensome, and to know when to tread lightly as a parent and when care and caution need to be taken.

In the spirit of giving and continuous learning that is the hallmark of all of Martine's work, you can stay up to date with new apps, new games, new alerts, technological advances, new strategies and new settings on her website. This book is the start of a wonderful journey into the world of digital parenting.

Enjoy the learning. You are in good hands.

Michael Grose
Founder, Parenting Ideas

INTRODUCTION

They don't know how to play outside.

They don't know how to use their imaginations.

They're overweight because they no longer run around and play.

They can't look people in the eye and communicate.

They don't know how to be bored.

They're lazy and expect everything in an instant.

These are just a few of the sweeping generalisations we hear from older generations and mainstream media about 'the kids of today'.

The irony being that it is these generalisations that are lazy.

It's easy to get a click-through to an article about kids being 'glued to their screens', 'preferring to stay indoors' and being 'more interested in likes and followers' than real-life interactions.

It's less easy to get a click-through to something about young people finding a way to thrive in the digital age.

Yet, I'm seeing and working with kids in the latter category every single day.

So the first thing I'd like to do is get one thing straight: the kids are going to be okay.

Your kid is going to be okay.

Why? Because you're reading this book. You've taken a proactive step towards better understanding the digital world they're living in.

THE CHALLENGE

Ten years ago, after combining a teaching background with a Masters in Counselling, I began working with kids and teenagers who were struggling with their wellbeing and family relationships.

While the problems those kids were presenting with varied, a common theme started to emerge: there seemed to be a huge divide between how parents and kids understood the digital world.

Parents were frustrated by their children's seeming reliance on digital devices.

Young people were frustrated that their parents' answer to any perceived problems was to simply curb or control their use of digital devices.

It became clear to me that in order for families to work together and live in harmony, parents needed to gain a greater perspective and understanding of the workings of the digital world their kids were playing in.

Gaining that perspective is difficult; however, when you consider the tendency of humans (augmented by the tendency of the media) to focus on the negatives.

Yes, there is a lot of bad stuff to be found in the world that has landed in the hands, laps and back pockets of our kids.

Yes, they are making contact with people who are undesirable.

Yes, they are being bullied, having photos taken and shared without consent, and missing out on opportunities because of online transgressions.

And then there are the contradictions.

On one hand, the online world can connect us. With the swipe of a screen or the touch of a button, we can engage in conversation with people thousands of kilometres away. But it can also disconnect us. Sometimes from those sitting only metres away from us.

How do we ensure
that our kids are
getting the very best
that technology has
to offer them?

It's a world that can both enlighten us with information, news and real-time events and fill our minds with untruths and heinous visual content.

It can be a place where a young person finds support, solace and friendship when they struggle to identify with their peers. But it can also be a place where a young person is bullied, stalked, abused or harassed when they struggle to identify with those peers.

And herein lies the challenge.

How do we ensure that our kids are getting the very best that technology has to offer them?

How do we ensure they're able to take advantage of the opportunities for learning and education, for collaborations and connections, for creativity and the endless possibilities?

How do we ensure they get all of that while steering clear of cyberbullying and sexting, predators and pornography, and the distractions and disturbances we hear about so often?

We need to be able to answer these questions because this world with all its technology is not going anywhere. Our kids are going to spend much of their lives immersed in it.

A PROACTIVE AND POSITIVE APPROACH

Here's what I know from what parents have told me, along with my own experience in parenting five boys (now aged between 8 and 19):

- We want our kids to feel safe and in control of their digital world.
- We want them to be able to navigate the risks in that world with confidence.
- We want them to grow, thrive, connect, create and collaborate despite those risks.

To do this, we have to be proactive in understanding the digital world a bit better ourselves.

Gone are the days where we can:

- ban access to an app just because we heard something bad happened on it
- dismissively say 'don't talk to people online if you don't want to get bullied'
- simply take away technology for days or weeks at a time in order to handle a transgression or counter a tantrum.

Technology and the devices are now so intricately and completely woven into the fabric of our lives, and more importantly into the lives of our children, that it would be neglectful to simply rely on these reactive measures to keep them safe and smart and in control.

It's totally appropriate to mandate:

- technology and device-free time
- developmental and age-appropriate boundaries and rules around what is suitable
- a culture of balanced play and learning so that they are educated and entertained from a variety of means.

But what about drumming into our kids the dangers of a life lived largely online? What about highlighting the bad things that happen to others in order to prevent them from happening to our own offspring? Is this type of 'preventive' teaching effective?

Increasingly, research and experience are showing us that simply lecturing about the dangers, or trying to ban and block the offending technology, does not always translate to long term, positive change.

A more proactive approach is to give our children experience, responsibility and the skills to be safe and smart. And the good news is, the way to do this is by doing what we're all doing already—being good, attentive and loving parents.

OUR ROLE AS PARENTS

We all want to raise great kids who are able to make the most of the opportunities presented by a digital world; who have the skills, thinking and behaviours necessary for facing the challenges this relatively new world presents.

To do that, we must remember that what it fundamentally means to be a parent and a child has not changed.

As a parent, our role is to keep our kids safe and protected, particularly when they are young. As they get older, our role is to nurture them and give them the skills to become independent and confident members of society by:

- setting good boundaries for them to operate within
- giving them safe places to test those boundaries and learn from the experience
- helping them develop the responsibility and skills to be safe and smart.

Being a child today hasn't really changed too much either.

Whilst they are young, they are happy to be protected by us and revel in the security we can provide.

As they get older; however, they want to start seeking out independence and will push against some of the boundaries that have been set up to protect them. They will want to find out who they are and where they belong. They will want to hang out with their mates and chat and flirt and share their lives.

The problem for us as parents today is that our kids are operating in a vastly different playground to the one we grew up in.

For younger kids, we need to better understand that playground so we can protect them and keep them safe whilst they play there.

As our kids get older, we need to be giving them the skills, thinking and behaviours to play safely in that playground when we're not there to hold their hand.

MOVING FROM FEAR TO EMPOWERMENT

There are certainly times I worry about the safety and wellbeing of young people in a digital world:

- when I speak to the little boy in Grade 2 who is playing Call of Duty and Grand Theft Auto, by himself, for many hours
- when I ask 9-year-olds if they are on Snapchat or Instagram and many little hands go up in the air

We don't want
our kids to be fearful,
overwhelmed and
anxious. We want
them to feel
confident, resilient
and empowered.

- when school principals, on an almost weekly basis, tell me there has been cyberbullying going on via a group chat, and the screenshots say its happening at 11 pm at night for these primary school-aged kids.

But I feel there are two distinct ways to deal with those worrying situations.

We can take the negative, fearful approach of focusing on all the dangers and trying to shut them all down.

Or we can do what we can to understand how the technology works and then use that knowledge to parent from a place of empowerment and positivity.

Experience has shown me that when a parent is fearful, overwhelmed, anxious and feeling powerless, some of those elements will rub off on the kids who are living those messages every day.

We don't want our kids to be fearful, overwhelmed, anxious and feeling powerless. We also don't want our kids left to their own devices (no pun intended) and with little input from parents who fear it is all too hard and not something they feel equipped to manage.

We want kids and parents to feel educated. We want them to feel confident, resilient and empowered to make the best choices they can. Or, at the very least, to continue to learn and grow and thrive, despite those challenges.

HOW THIS BOOK WILL WORK

This book is a culmination of all the teaching, writing and conversations I have had with my readers, parents, students and teachers over the last decade.

I'm going to start by debunking some myths before sharing my thoughts on how to decide whether your child is ready for a device. A key part of using a device and participating in the online world safely is to develop critical thinking. Chapter Three offers tips about mindful content consumption.

Chapter Four will help you educate your child on the digital footprint they are creating and then things will get a little heavy. I'll talk about recognising grooming and the behaviour of online predators. Then I'll share how to deal with both the real and confected dramas of social media before going into the recognition and management of cyberbullying.

From there, things get lighter as I share the good that can be accomplished with the help of social media, how to manage screen time effectively, before covering how to game in a healthy fashion.

In my 10 years working with parents and children to effectively manage and communicate about this online world, I've come to see that while there is a lot of advice that is specific to apps and certain situations, there are certain strategies that are timeless. For the most part, this book shares more timeless approaches.

For advice and strategies that are specific to an app or moment in time, my website is the best place to visit. That's where I share more specific or time-sensitive information in addition to the most recent research findings. New apps, new games, new alerts, technological advances, new strategies, new settings: all this information on my website, in conjunction with the more evergreen information in this book will allow you to have the right conversations with your kids and put in place the best practices for your family.

I will also note that whilst this book offers some ideas around boundaries and use of devices, I'm not here to give you every rule that you should implement. Each family's situation is very different. Each individual child and their needs can also be vastly different.

That's why my main goal with this book is to enable you and your children to have conversations that move you towards understanding and perspective, conversations that will help you come together with your own set of boundaries and strategies to work within your family circumstances.

To facilitate this, at the end of each chapter, I challenge you to ponder a few of the issues covered and question your own thinking. I also have some discussion questions to help you broach some of these topics that may be relevant to your child.

CHAPTER 1

··

DEBUNKING some of the key myths and mindsets about the online world

··························

In any industry, there are myths that arise, usually due to media attention. Before you know it, those myths turn into 'conventional wisdom' and from there quickly become entrenched beliefs.

This is certainly true when it comes to parenting in the digital age. So let's take some time now to put some of those myths and beliefs under the microscope.

MYTH 1: THINGS MOVE SO FAST, IT'S IMPOSSIBLE TO KEEP UP

Yes, it's true that technology seems to be evolving at the speed of light.

And it can feel quite disconcerting when it seems our kids know more about technology than we do. Upload, download, share, like, Airdrop, Snapstreak, emoji—

they're not just across all these terms but can also fix grandma's phone every time she locks herself out and they have the skills and technical 'know-how' to navigate their way around every gaming console or smart device they come across. The ease at which they do all these things can quickly leave us feeling 'left behind'.

But it's important to remember that this world of devices and technology is all our kids have ever known. They've grown up with all these things so their skills in this arena are almost innate.

What they're not born with; however, is the ability to understand the idiosyncrasies of a world that is so connected, public and magnified. A world that requires an understanding of:

- human relationships and behaviours
- consequences and repercussions
- the challenges of a very public journey through adolescence.

Their developing brains and bodies and their quest for independence and identity can be a cauldron of trouble when it all happens in a big public internet melting pot.

As parents, we don't need to have intimate knowledge of every site they visit or every app they are using. All we need to know are the sorts of things technology is capable of and the ways that kids are using it.

And we already know this. (If you don't, this book will help.) Which leaves us to focus our efforts on helping them develop the habits, behaviours, skills and thinking they need to be safe and smart wherever they find themselves online.

MYTH 2: MY CHILD IS TOO YOUNG FOR ME TO HAVE TO WORRY

The average age a child first swipes an iPad is about 12 months of age.

The average household in Australia has around seven internet-enabled devices.

Even if you're not a particularly techy, screen-filled family, chances are you are using some form of mobile technology in your daily lives. Most people are sharing their child's lives online, some even before they are delivered via their ultrasound pictures. Many birth announcements are made via a Facebook feed. Toddlers are Skyping their grandparents overseas, using devices to watch Peppa Pig, listening to audiobooks or playing Alphabet Lotto on the iPad. Some of the most downloaded apps are in the toddler and preschool sections of the online app stores. And even if your child doesn't spend time on technology, they are certainly watching the role that it plays in your life.

We cannot take
a 'set and forget'
approach to using
internet filters and
privacy settings.

Regardless of a child's age, we need to start thinking about how technology will be incorporated into their lives.

MYTH 3: FILTERS WILL KEEP MY CHILD SAFE

Yes, it's absolutely essential to have good internet filters and effectively managed privacy settings. But we cannot take a 'set and forget' approach to using these tools.

Kids will have playdates with kids whose families have not been so diligent. They may find themselves on a bus, in the park or even at school sitting with a kid whose device is unprotected and who willingly shares all manner of content with them. Many devices are not protected once they log in to the free WiFi at the local cafe. Many kids are also pretty good at changing settings and getting around filters.

So, whilst we can certainly continue to do everything we can to protect and manage the devices being used in our homes, we cannot afford to leave it at that. Despite our best efforts, our kids will almost certainly be exposed to content and people that are certainly not in their best interest.

MYTH 4: PREVENTING ACCESS WILL KEEP MY CHILD SAFE

I've had many conversations with parents who are overwhelmed by the possibility of what their child could be exposed to. They've heard all the horror stories, clicked on the alarming headlines and been freaked out by situations other young people have found themselves in online. And their solution has been prevention by way of banning and blocking everything.

Experience has taught me that this is rarely a workable solution.

Kids are going to hang out where their mates are hanging out. Kids are good at creating second accounts for the social networks you have insisted on having the password to.

It's also important to note that they are often using social networks as an important lifeline to strengthen connections, enhance relationships, manage social events and participate in society as they know it.

Now I'm not advocating that you let your youngsters have free rein on any social media site they so desire. But a core goal of this book is to share ways we can help our kids stay safe and make good decisions without having to constantly try and shut everything down and relentlessly monitor every place they visit.

MYTH 5: SMARTPHONES ARE MAKING US DEPRESSED

We've all seen the headlines:

> *Mobile phones are causing depression.*
>
> *Child suicide rates rise with device use.*
>
> *Smartphones have destroyed a generation.*

Yes, there are many statistics to be found correlating increases in depression and anxiety with the increase in mobile device use. But it's important to know that correlation does not necessarily denote causation.

Young people might be self-reporting more these days about having depression and anxiety; the definition of what actually constitutes screen time is very convoluted, and not all screen time is equal.

Can depression and anxiety be exacerbated or caused by online experiences? Yes.

Are mobile devices causing depression and anxiety? Current research cannot categorically say that.

Thankfully there are many researchers going much deeper than the shallows of these headlines and arriving at far more nuanced and complex theories about depression in kids and the relationship to phones. They are now seeing a need for better data collection, more specific questions, a greater look at other factors of the individual and the environment. They've identified the need to enlist the help of the big tech companies who have the most drilled down data about how kids are using the devices.

The links between devices and mental health is certainly an important one. But let's understand the implication of making rash generalisations that will not serve our young people well and may well be masking other factors that also need to be addressed.

MYTH 6: ALL SCREEN TIME IS EQUAL

One of the greatest takeaways I hope you get from this book is the ability to look more critically at exactly what our kids are doing on the screens and to understand that lumping screen time under the one banner is unhelpful.

In fact, because the ways we use screens—the different types of games, interactions, experiences, tasks, intentions and outcomes—are all so different, it's likely the term 'screen time' will soon become obsolete.

Think of all the different ways a child could make use of 30 minutes of 'screen time':

- setting up a 'GoFundMe' page to save koalas
- watching cat videos on YouTube

- exploring the latest satellite vision on the NASA website
- cyberbullying someone on a social media feed
- downloading music whilst painting a landscape
- watching pornography
- composing a song
- crushing some candy.

The experiences and effects of the above are certainly not equal in the way they attribute to the development, learning and wellbeing of your child.

MYTH 7: DEVICES ARE CURBING CREATIVITY

Another common concern of parents is that having so much entertainment on hand (via screens) compromises their child's ability to be creative and let their imaginations run free.

This may be true in some cases. But in many cases, advances in technology have allowed kids to explore creativity in vastly different ways than before and possibly opened up creativity to children who would otherwise not be such willing participants:

- a well thought out design or creation may be created in an art or drawing app

Devices give kids
freedom to explore
classroom topics in
a manner that is
meaningful to them.

- a song may be recorded on a music creating app
- photos and videos may become movies or animations.

I have also been witness to the many wonderful ways devices have allowed children in a classroom setting to engage more fully with a topic (in a way that still fulfils learning outcomes) because devices give kids freedom to explore those topics in a manner that is meaningful to them.

- I've seen them create online books, poems, songs to music, animations, and recorded interviews.

- I've seen kids create a pseudo-Facebook page for the famous person in history they're studying and use that exercise to highlight their daily life and get a feel for their challenges, where they hang out, what they read, who their friends are and what they wear.

- I've also seen a classroom create Snapchat stories for the day in the life of a soldier in World War I.

For many kids, the above is far more engaging and requires more creativity than writing an essay on the life of their historical subject.

Things to ponder

- How would I have used the technology of today if it was available to me when I was young?

- What role does technology play in our lives at the moment? Am I comfortable with the message this sends to my child?

- How does my child hear me talk about technology?

- What are some of the areas that I believe will require greater boundaries, effort and input when it comes to navigating a digital world with my child?

Conversations to have with your kids

- What are the main differences you see about how we as parents grew up and the way children today are growing up?

- What do you think are the positive things about growing up with such ready access to the online world?

- What are the negative aspects of growing up with that access to the online world?

- What are some of the biggest challenges you've faced in being part of that online world?
- What challenges do you foresee for yourself or your peers in the near future?
- Do you feel confident to handle those challenges?
- Do you feel supported to get help should you need it?

CHAPTER 2

....

DECIDING whether your child is ready for their own device

....

One of the most common questions I hear from parents is *When should my child get their own device for the first time?*

Is it when all their mates get one?

When they are starting out on public transport?

Spending more time home alone?

Is it when the school insists they need one?

When they turn a certain age?

Like many of our challenges today, the answer is not always simple. (And let's also remember that handing over a device doesn't mean you also have to hand over the reins to every social media, game or app that is out there. There are ways to use a device without giving access to places you don't want your child to visit and content you don't want them to view.)

FOUR KEY THINGS TO CONSIDER

There are four things I want you to consider before deciding to give your child a device of their own. These aren't meant to be scary or off-putting and make you decide your child should never get near any device ever. Rather, they are designed to ensure that when you hand a device to your child, it's with your eyes wide open. And to ensure that you understand your role here is like with any other parenting issue—to monitor and keep the lines of communication open so you are able to support them through challenges and help them develop skills they can call on for the rest of their lives.

1. The young brain's cognitive development

Part of being a young child is having a young brain that is growing and developing and being nurtured by the experiences provided to it. Young brains are a long way from where they need to be to process many of the situations they find themselves in when engaging with platforms, games and apps developed by adults for adults. Things such as impulse control, ethical thinking and reactive decision making are not yet developed in young people to the level that many of these networks and games require.

The complex thinking needed to make the most accurate assumptions about the connections they make and the content they devour, needs to be part of their education from the moment they start hanging out online. Otherwise, cognitively, socially and emotionally, they are just not ready.

2. That age is an arbitrary measure

'Reaching a certain age' often appears to be a logical answer to the question of whether a child is ready for their own device. And '13 years of age' often seems to be this age. Most likely because this is the magic number the majority of social platforms state is the age their platform can be used from.

Dig a little deeper; however, and you'll find out how arbitrary this age constraint is. Most social networks only have it because they need to comply with the USA's COPPA law (Children's Online Privacy Protection Act). This law states that it is illegal for companies to obtain certain information and data from any child under the age of 13 without parental consent. To escape any jurisdictional breaches and avoid legal minefields, the creators of the apps simply make them 13+. Furthermore, this restriction is an advisory category, not a legal one.

The reality is, there is a lot to hanging out online that is not addressed by birthday milestones. You only need to witness adults operating in irrational, unethical and/ or downright mean ways online to see the truth of this.

Age is a poor
determinant for
deciding whether
your child should be
granted their own
device or not.

So age is a poor determinant for deciding whether your child should be granted their own device or not.

3. The need for social and emotional maturity

Aside from the cognitive and thinking skills required, there is certainly an element of social and emotional maturity that one needs to play safely and well online.

Before we can expose our kids to the rigours of online conversations, group chats, interactions, innuendos and battles, it's better that they have first developed the social skills and emotional intelligence that come from surviving the friendship squabbles and schoolyard shenanigans of the real world.

How do we do the latter? We need to give them ample time to hang with friends. Unstructured. Not always interrupting. Not always solving their problems. Not always breaking apart the fights (unless of course there is blood or broken bones). We need to talk with them about how they handled certain situations at a play date, in the school ground or on the sporting field. Have they had enough time just testing things out? Seeing how to treat people? Getting an understanding of how they want to be treated?

Before we hand them a device, or an email account for a social networking app or set them up on a server to play

Minecraft online, we need to consider whether we have given them enough real world opportunities to have a few falls, endure a few bumps and scratches, and find the resilience to get back up and have another go, move on, mend friendships, assert themselves and continue playing.

Confidence in, or at least a good understanding of, your child's social and emotional maturity is a better measure than age.

4. The realities of the online world

When we connect online we are not only connecting with peers and friendship groups. Many times we are exposing ourselves and being exposed to the whole gamut of humans and their differing beliefs, values, backgrounds, experiences and circumstances. Add to that, anonymity, the bravado of sitting behind a keyboard, the ease of social media platforms to have a voice, and we have a whole melting pot of human interaction that can be anything from kind, humble and supportive, to abusive, violent and downright heinous.

Everything in real life is amplified in the online world. The better we understand this, the better we can effectively support our kids in playing and engaging safely there.

SOME SIMPLE STEPS AND GUIDELINES

1. Start with some boundaries

It is important we are the ones in the driver's seat when kids are starting out. The pull of devices is such that they need help to regulate some of their behaviours and form good habits. Think of the control you exert over what your kids eat. You don't give them free rein. Instead you give them a balanced and healthy diet and only allow treats at certain times. This builds strong habits that allow them to make good choices as they get older.

The same applies with devices. It is important to set boundaries that fit with your values and lifestyles and the needs of your child.

2. Let the leash out slowly

Once you've set up some strong boundaries and your child has gotten used to the role technology will play in their lives, you can slowly let the leash out a little. You can give them some autonomy over how they spend their time. Once they have a realisation of all the things they need to be healthy, and an understanding of what is important to them in their world, then we can give them a greater rein to understand how their tech use is going to affect those choices. This is not always easy and can happen at very different times. Some kids can work with technology in ways that they manage well on their own and so we can relax a little with some of our rules. Others; however, may take a lot longer to find that ability and we may need to continue to use our boundaries to help them maintain some balance before letting them make all those decisions.

3. Monitor then mentor

When kids are young or starting out on a social network it's important that we closely monitor what they are doing. Remember, their brain development is often not at the point that is needed to make independent decisions without some education and guidance.

So we support their play, learning and socialisation by keeping tabs of:

- who they are talking to
- whether or not they have an understanding of how to determine who they are talking to
- where their cognitive ability sits with regard to making decisions that could affect their safety and wellbeing.

As they grow in this understanding and thinking we can continue to talk to them about their online experiences but steer away from monitoring as such and instead become their mentor. Lead by example and learn from each other. Of course if you see red flags that things are not going so well, then you may well have to once again become more involved.

WATCHING FOR RED FLAGS

Despite our best efforts there can be times when kids find themselves in situations that do require further monitoring or delving in order to determine that their safety and wellbeing is not at risk. We need to be on the lookout for red flags that may suggest our kids are experiencing something online that is doing them harm. Things such as:

- spending increasing amounts of time online and doing so in a secretive manner

- a refusal to participate in activities they would usually enjoy

- no longer enjoying the company of their real-life friendships

- becoming moody and withdrawn (difficult to tell though with some teenagers).

When kids are young or starting out on a social network it's important that we closely monitor what they are doing.

Ultimately, it's important to trust your gut. You know your child well and if something doesn't feel right with them, then you need to listen to that instinct and take action to find out more about what is going on. Then get them the help that is needed should this be the case.

....

Things to ponder

....

- Do I feel my child has the emotional maturity to handle conflict or unwanted attention?

- Do I feel they have the cognitive development to make informed decisions about who people really are, the content they are consuming and the information they are sharing?

- Can they look adequately ahead to have an understanding of the consequences for their actions on their reputation or the feelings of others?

- How much am I going to monitor my child's device use? Will this affect areas of trust?

- What are the signs to look for that will determine their readiness or not for wherever they are hanging out?

- Is the idea that everyone else is using it a good enough excuse to let my child have access?
- What can I put in place to ensure I am maintaining control until I feel they have the maturity and skills to be more autonomous with their online activity?

....

Conversations to have with your kids

....

- Do you feel comfortable in coming to me should something upset you?
- Who else is someone you could turn to if you felt scared or uncomfortable?
- What level of parental involvement do you think is fair when starting out with a device or on social media?
- What are the things you think the technology may take you away from doing?
- When are the times that using technology is not going to be helpful for you to achieve the things you need to achieve and the things you would like to spend your time on?

CHAPTER 3

....

TEACHING critical thinking when it comes to content consumption

....

One of the most crucial skills we can teach young people when it comes to helping them navigate the online world is how to critically evaluate the content they consume. As we are inundated with copious amounts of new content every second of every day, the ability to determine the relevance, validity, truthfulness and safety of those videos, photos, memes and articles becomes increasingly difficult and problematic.

Here are some of the challenges we face in teaching our kids those critical thinking skills they need.

CHALLENGE 1: THE SHEER VOLUME OF CONTENT

When I was growing up my information came from the books and magazines I would read. It came from television, radio and newspapers and the people in my immediate circles. The news was a 30-minute nightly bulletin.

It's safe to say the content we all consume today is far more pervasive and invasive. Every day we are saturated by news, videos, articles, memes, photos, snaps, messages, and emails. We can spend countless hours scrolling and swiping our way through streams and streams of information.

CHALLENGE 2: THE LACK OF FACT-CHECKING

When a video is uploaded to YouTube or a meme is circulated via social media, there are no checks on facts or statistics or appropriateness for a particular audience before it is allowed to go online and be viewed by the rest of the world.

As mentioned, our kids have access to such a large range of information. And a huge proportion of that information has not been assessed or appraised as to its worthiness, truthfulness, safety and value to their physical, cognitive, social or emotional health and wellbeing.

CHALLENGE 3: EXPOSURE TO ATROCITIES

One of the biggest downsides to the lack of regulation thus far is the exposure to violence and inappropriate videos. As we have seen many times, heinous crimes and atrocities videoed are often live-streamed and played out on the feeds of all, including countless unsuspecting or possibly curious young people. 'Dares' and 'challenges' also find their way onto multiple social networks as the next cool thing to do to get oneself noticed, join a group or just gain some likes. Past challenges such as the 'cinnamon challenge', the 'Tide pod challenge' and the 'super gluing your lips challenge' have exposed the dangerous lengths some people will go to in order to gain notoriety or just to feel like they belong. The popularity of live video has seen many young people go to dangerous, even fatal, lengths to capture a video that ensures they stand out in the crowd.

CHALLENGE 4: ONLINE PORNOGRAPHY IS PROLIFIC

There are many things about the online world I have happily moved along with, despite a little nostalgia for days gone by. But this element of the global, exaggerated and magnified world of the internet is one that causes me concern.

A huge proportion of online information has not been assessed or appraised as to its truthfulness and value.

Long gone are those days of young boys saving their pennies to buy Playboy magazines, share them around and hide them under their beds. The images may certainly have been eye-opening to the young adolescent, but it's fair to say they had nothing on the substantially more graphic depictions their little minds are now being exposed to via online porn sites.

Pornography is made by adults. For adults. A visual interpretation of fantasy. And for the most part, adults have the ability to differentiate between fantasy and reality. Our kids don't.

They need to be made aware that there will be images they see online that may make them feel confused, disgusted or uncomfortable. They can be described as rude or yucky or whatever language you think they may use. They also need to know that they will not be in trouble should they see these images, but we do want to do what we can to ensure they don't become regular viewing.

THE NEED FOR BETTER CRITICAL THINKING SKILLS

When children are left to their own devices, they have to do a lot of thinking on their own.

- There is no one to tell them that following this person or this social media feed isn't going to do their self-esteem any good.

- There is no one to pose the question *Is this a biased opinion? Or even advertising?*
- There is no one to say *Those stats on the meme were made up.*
- There is no one to tell us *This could be dangerous* or *You need a parent's consent.*
- There is no one reminding us of the extraordinary skills many Photoshop users have and the lengths many people go to get the perfect image.
- They may not have anyone interpreting the violence that popped up on their feed that was shared via a group chat.
- There may not be anyone helping them make sense of the pornography they viewed and how continuing to view it on a regular basis could have ramifications for their future relationships and for their expectations of themselves and others.

They will need to come to these conclusions themselves. Every time they come across a photo or video, an article, a blog post, a tweet or a meme, they must be able to determine the relevance, benefits, accuracy and importance of consuming that media. Here are some tools and topics you can use to help your child think more critically.

STRATEGY 1: CURATE A MORE BALANCED VIEW OF THE WORLD

If you're like many people these days, you get most of your news from your social media feed. The problem with this is that we tend to follow the same sort of people, read the same sort of articles, and adhere to the same sort of beliefs. This narrows our view of the world considerably. It also means we don't quite understand that the news and opinions we're getting in our own feeds might be vastly different from the ones another person is getting.

In the same way the above is happening for adults, so too is happening for kids. While it's not intentional, the views and opinions they are exposed to are overly curated to match their existing beliefs.

So, how do we counter this?

The main thing we can do is follow media outlets that are not necessarily aligned with everything we believe in. This can be confronting and challenging but is necessary for ensuring you're not operating in an echo chamber where opinions and beliefs are accepted as fact simply because they're in line with how you think already.

Once you have experienced the challenges of following these kinds of media outlets yourself and found a way to process that conflicting information in a critical fashion, you can then pass those skills on to your kids.

STRATEGY 2: DIFFERENTIATE BETWEEN FAKE AND FALSE VERSUS TRUE AND HELPFUL

The term 'fake news' emerged to cover information that, for whatever reason, cannot be viewed as trustworthy.

It may be where untrue content is deliberately and maliciously created and shared in order to spread disinformation.

It may be the skewing of news and events to support an underlying agenda.

It may be the proliferation of misinformation as a result of limited fact-checking, either due to time limitations or the lack of ethical practices by online blogs and websites who are not subjected to the same constraints of traditional media outlets.

Advancing technology and the greater speed at which we do just about everything, has led us to impart greater importance on getting things done fast, as opposed to done right. Many political parties, groups and individuals have taken to social media sharing to get their message out, win over a vote, sway those on the cusp or bolster the beliefs of those already on board. Whilst spinning stories, lies and deceit is nothing new, it is safe to say the speed and extent to which they reach their targets, is unprecedented.

As with the above strategy, we adults have to make the adjustment first. We need to work on our verification and validation skills. We need to understand the behaviours that lead to media outlets spreading fake news. Once we're across that ourselves, we can coach our children in processing that information effectively.

STRATEGY 3: STEER KIDS AWAY FROM UNREGULATED CONTENT

When kids are young we can set up filters that ensure they are not exposed to violence, pornography and other content that they simply do not have the cognitive and emotional development to process.

We can also steer them away from unregulated sites like YouTube and Google, and towards quality online publishers like ABC Kids and Netflix Kids that are both kid-specific, and not open to the public to add their own content. Additionally, games that cost money are generally going to be of a higher quality than free

We adults have to
make the adjustment
first. We need
to work on our
verification and
validation skills.

games that serve up advertisements, many of which will be related to gambling. You can also turn off in-app purchases.

····································
Things to ponder
····································

- Through whose eyes and ears is my child viewing the world?
- Does my child have a grasp of the nuances of what is fake, real, opinion or advertising?
- Is the media they are consuming any more or less relevant than books or news broadcasts (i.e the media we consumed in our day)?
- Am I prepared to have discussions (no matter how embarrassing and awkward) about pornography with my child?
- Do I think I would know if my child had viewed pornography?
- What if my child views a violent act that is live-streamed? How will I support them through that? Have I thought about how I explain the bad things they may be exposed to?

Conversations to have with your kids

Some of these questions will naturally arise when researching for school projects, looking up things online as a family or even researching a holiday destination:

- Why should we look for more than one source when researching something online?

- What clues can we look for that something is advertising or trying to sell us a product or service?

- How do language and imagery determine how we feel about content?

- How can we check facts/data/research when consuming content online?

- What types of websites or media outlets may be more trustworthy than others?

- Would there be warnings on the content you consume if it was on television or mainstream media? (Warnings about age restrictions, nudity, violence, drug use etc.)

- Have you ever seen anything online that made you afraid, confused or you knew wasn't created for your eyes? What can you do if you happen to see this again?

- Do you have someone you would be able to talk to if you saw something online you didn't understand or was threatening or didn't feel right?

Conversations to have with your OLDER kids

- Do you understand how real-life relationships are different from the relationships portrayed in online pornography?
- What are some of the expectations for both boys and girls that are presented in online pornography?
- What do you understand about consent? How does consent affect what we share online and what we experience in the real world?
- What are the gender stereotypes that are often portrayed in pornography?

CHAPTER 4

....

UNDERSTANDING
our digital footprint

....

Our digital footprint is quite simply the information we leave behind every time we go online. This trail of people, content, likes, shares, searches and interactions all begin to form a picture and tell a story about who we are, how we see the world and how we are being represented to the rest of the world.

The sorts of things that contribute to our digital footprint are:

- the people we connect with, follow or friend
- the articles, memes or videos that we read, view, circulate and share
- the sites we visit
- the terms we search
- the games we play
- the networks we are part of

- the language we use
- the ways we behave
- the ways we interact and connect and how we respond to others
- the information we share
- the information we keep private
- the places we shop
- our likes and our dislikes
- what we respond to.

The digital footprint we are creating really does become a reflection of who we are. While we don't want to completely alarm kids, it's important they know that everything they do online has the potential to be scrutinised and judged, and could ultimately affect their future chances of employment. Whilst they will be contributing enormous amounts of data and mistakes will certainly happen, it is important to remember employers frequently Google people first when considering them for a position. There are also things they could be doing right now that may be affected by their digital footprint. Things like wanting to be a school captain, sports captain, get the lead in a play, or even getting a babysitting job.

If our kids are seen to be doing the wrong thing online, disrespecting themselves or others, they may find these footprints follow them around and in turn mean they may not get those coveted roles.

UNDERSTANDING WHAT A 'LIKE' SAYS

I was once at a school where a young person took a photo of the maths teacher and posted it to Instagram (a private account separate to the one their mum and dad had access to). The caption on the photo alluded to their dislike of said teacher and the subject in general. The photo received many likes and comments from their peers.

A mother of another child happened to be checking what her child was 'liking', came across this photo and took it to the school. Subsequently, all those kids from the school who 'liked' the photo were reprimanded and given a suspension.

This might sound like a harsh penalty for students who had neither taken the photo or commented, but merely 'liked' it. It was a reminder that when you 'like' something, whether you realise it or not, you are saying, 'I agree with this and endorse what the message represents'.

Which is why we all need to be mindful of what we like, share and comment on, as we never really know who is watching and may well find ourselves 'guilty by association'.

When you 'like' something, you are saying, 'I agree with this and endorse what the message represents'.

TAKING CONTROL OF OUR DIGITAL FOOTPRINT

There are two things we can't control in the online world.

The first is that we can't control what people will do with our content.

Regardless of what privacy settings we use, or who we originally send something to, once we put something online we literally give up all control over what happens to those words, images, videos, comments, emails and text messages.

Take the example of even a simple text message between two people. The person at the other end can forward on the message. They can copy and paste it to another network. They can take a screenshot of it and save it for future use.

The second thing we can't control is the behaviour of other people.

We cannot control the things other people say.

We cannot control what they share—the images they post, the comments they make, the videos they circulate.

Here's what we can control.

We can control what *we* put out into the online world.

For this, I share a simple rule with young people: if you can think of just one person in the whole world you don't want to see this, then don't hit send.

We can also control *how we respond* to nasty people.

This is not always easy and can take some practice, but it is such a critical mindset to have today. In my work with students, we often look at conversations and interactions that occur online and role-play how the fallout can often be detrimental to both your wellbeing and your digital footprint.

Let's take this interaction as an example:

> **Lily:** I just love the new song by (insert favourite pop star).
>
> **Bella:** OMG, are you kidding? Worst song ever. No taste ... get a life.

I then ask the kids how they think Lily should respond. We come up with options such as:

A. Ignore the comment.

B. Reply with something like *No stress, we all have different taste.*

C. Reply with something like *You think I've got no taste? You have no idea, loser.*

We then discuss how these different responses would play out.

For the record both A and B are fine.

If one chooses C; however, we soon come to the conclusion that we will most likely end up in a sledging match where no one is going to win and you are going to spend a good deal of time, and emotional energy trying to both deal with the fallout and come up with bigger and better responses.

For the record, many adults are not very good at this and often head down the path of C. (One only needs to read the comment sections of popular blogs or media outlets to see how many adults have not learnt the skill of knowing when to abort an online conversation!)

I frequently remind the kids I work with that focusing on the best response for the wellbeing of both ourselves and others, as well as our digital footprint, allows us to ascertain whether or not a response is even warranted, and if so how we can best word our response to ensure we are not creating further drama and turmoil.

PRIVACY AND DATA

Back in 1967, Alan Westin, in his book *Privacy and Freedom*, described privacy as:

> *The claim of individuals, groups or institutions to determine for themselves, when, how and to what extent information about them is communicated to others.*

Still relevant today, his work led to the transformation of many laws concerning privacy. In more recent years; however, he conceded that laws alone can no longer determine our privacy. Rather we need a combination of legal, technological and social fixes as well as constant education as to our rights, and our self-determination of these rights.

Danah Boyd, author of *It's Complicated: the social lives of networked teens* notes that in the past, you had to work hard to be public. Now, you must work hard to be private. The tables have definitely turned.

With regard to data, it's important to acknowledge that everything we do online is tracked and traced and oftentimes bought and sold. There are generally three ways our data is collected online:

1. **Data Given:** This is data we knowingly hand over. The photos we share. The comments we make. The goods we buy. All the data we contribute every time we participate online.

2. **Data Traces:** Data left behind from what we have given becomes data traces of our online participation. This is usually less knowingly handed over because it is captured by tracking technologies such as cookies, location data, web tracking etc.

3. **Inferred Data:** This is the data that comes from analysing the first two above. Our data given and the traces left behind allow for analysis to create and profile our online behaviours. This may then play out in the pages and pictures we are shown, corporations and companies we are advertised to and the people and places that may be suggested to us as a good fit.

Many young people today simply accept that the dress they put in their cart but didn't buy will continue to come up in their advertising feeds. They know that when they search for 'Bali holidays', they will continue to be bombarded with holiday deals. Others see these things as ranging from mildly creepy to major fraud.

16 TIPS FOR MAINTAINING SOME SEMBLANCE OF PRIVACY AND DATA CONTROL

1. Use privacy settings and check them regularly for changes. Many settings are not private by default and we need to physically go in and make the changes to turn on or toggle off.

2. Install third-party software. If you visit **themodernparent.net/resources** you will find the different products I recommend for limiting the sites you can access and the information that can

It's important to
acknowledge that
everything we do
online is tracked and
traced and oftentimes
bought and sold.

be shared. Once again we still need to be careful with what we share and the information we give away, but the privacy systems and software can be a good backstop.

3. Always set up two-factor authentication to ensure your social networks are not easily hacked. This can be done for most of your online accounts and is the best way to add that extra layer of protection to prevent other people from accessing your account and data. (Two-factor authentication essentially means you need a password and a code each time you log in which will be sent to another device of your choosing.)

4. Ask permission before posting photos of others, especially if you are unsure of their views of online sharing. And if you don't want photos of your kids shared by others, be sure to say so when you know photos are being taken.

5. Ask photos to be removed if concerned. If it is a particularly sensitive photo that has been shared without your consent and is causing you hurt or embarrassment, first ask the person to take it down. If they don't, you can then ask the social network or platform the image is found on. If they do nothing after 48 hours, in Australia you can go to the Office of the eSafety Commissioner (**esafety.gov.au**). They have the ability to override the networks and have the image removed.

6. Post personal photos to select groups or friends online. If you don't want photos shared with all

your friends and all of their friends, you can create smaller, more relevant groups to share your photos with. You can also set up Facebook so that you are alerted and required to grant permission when you are tagged in someone else's photo.

7. Do the right checks before handing over private information or credit card details. If the product sounds too good to be true, that may well be the case. Read the reviews of others who have purchased.

8. Be wary of winning anything online. Once again, if it sounds too good to be true, it usually is. Teach your kids to automatically click the cross and close down pop-ups. Scamwatch can be a good resource for getting verification and the heads up on the latest scams.

9. Consume content with a healthy dose of scepticism. We don't want to become complete cynics, but we must view this world with a critical eye that forces us to question the validity of what we are consuming. We need to ask ourselves the questions:

   • How do I know this is true?

   • What information do I need to back this up?

   • What research have they used?

   • Why was this written or produced?

   • Who is the author or publisher?

10. Look for clues that the page or person you are following is the real profile/page for that person. Does the page for the large corporation or the superstar pop star have 34 followers? If so, it's not going to be the real one. Ask yourself:

- What do I need to know to prove they are who they say they are?

- What other information may I need before I proceed?

11. Shop from secure sites. Look for the padlocks. Read the reviews. Ensure the site is encrypted with Secure Sockets Layer (SSL) which will mean the URL will begin with HTTPS rather than just HTTP.

12. Be wary of logging in to public WiFi networks.

13. Understand what your new toys can find out about you. Google Home and even baby monitors can collect a whole lot of stuff about you without you realising. That's not to say there will be any negative impact. But it's good to know what you are handing over.

14. Learn to know the difference between fact, opinion and advertising. Looking for clues as to whether something is true and factual, or possibly trying to encourage you to purchase something or hand over money is a crucial skill today.

15. Understand how the games and networks your kids play on work. Reviews on specific games and networks can be found on my website.

16. Trust your gut. Listen to that feeling in your stomach that suggests this may not be what it's cracked up to be. Get your kids to listen to that feeling in their stomach that says:

- This person may not be who they say they are.
- This person doesn't actually need this information about me.
- This person may well be lying about what they are going to do with this photo.

The above list is by no means exhaustive and will not provide 100% protection from data breaches and oversharing. But it's a good place to start to ensure you are doing what you can and teaching your children to do what they can to remain in control of the information and data that is being shared about you online.

Things to ponder

- How is my child's view of privacy likely to be different to mine?
- Are kids different today with what they share or do they just have a different means of sharing?
- How am I affecting my child's digital footprint?
- In what ways am I teaching them about taking control of how they are presented online?

Conversations to have with your kids

- What sorts of information should you never need to put online? (These responses will obviously differ with different age groups.)
- Do you know what happens to your data when you share information online?
- What sorts of steps can you take to keep things private?
- Can you think of anything that you are doing right now or would like to do in the near future that might be affected by your online behaviour?

Trust your gut. Listen
to that feeling in
your stomach that
suggests this may not
be what it's cracked
up to be.

- Do you feel comfortable with what you share being viewed, commented on or shared by people you don't know?

- What parts of your life would you like to maintain control over in terms of keeping it offline? What steps will you need to take to ensure this is maintained?

- Are you comfortable letting friends know the things you don't want to be shared about you online?

CHAPTER 5

··

RECOGNISING grooming, online predators and image-based abuse

··

Grooming is when a paedophile intentionally connects with a young person with the goal of:

- having the young person send images or videos online, or
- meeting up with the young person in real life with the intention of committing a sexual offence.

Grooming can be done online using any social network, any messaging app or any game.

Like all predators, those grooming young people online work very hard and in very clever ways to win over the trust of their victims. They usually begin by 'friending' or 'following' someone on a social network, messaging service or game. From there, they build relationships of trust to create a platform from which they can then manipulate that person into doing things for their own means and enjoyment. The types of relationships they can create include:

- a boyfriend/girlfriend type relationship where the victim is made to feel they are loved by this person.
- a mentor-type relationship where they start off by teaching or motivating the victim to achieve something.

Two difficulties with identifying and preventing grooming are:

- the predator might be someone known to the child (either a friend of the family or a family member)
- the way grooming mimics positive, loving or caring relationships.

Online predators work on building trust to the point that they have significant power over the young person, who then often finds themselves starting to question their level of trust of other people in their lives (the ones they usually should be trusting). This then allows the predator to coerce the young person to do things either as a way to strengthen that trust or through blackmail or the fear of others finding out.

I have seen countless situations where young people have been scammed by people claiming to have images they have stolen by hacking into their devices or by taking photos via their webcam and then using these as threats to share with all the people in their contact list if they don't accede to the demands. This can be sending more pictures or videos or it can be for the purpose of making money as a blackmail situation.

HOW TO RECOGNISE GROOMING BEHAVIOUR

It can generally be said that kids in vulnerable positions, with low self-esteem, who are socially or geographically isolated from others, can more easily fall victim to online abuse.

But, ultimately, it is very difficult to recognise when a child is being groomed.

We can look out for signs of withdrawal, spending long hours on a device or being secretive about their time online. We can be alert to them receiving unexplained gifts or obtaining online money or gaming credits. We can pay attention if they get defensive when approached about their online behaviours.

We can also help our kids to be aware of tactics like:

- Flattery (You look gorgeous, I could help you with a modelling career, I can't believe all the boys/girls are not swooning over you.)

It is very difficult
to recognise when
a child is being
groomed.

- The offer of money or gifts (I can get you tickets to your favourite rock band. I can help you make money really easily.)
- Sympathy (You seem really upset, how can I help? It seems like you don't have a lot of great friends right now.)

The most important thing to understand; however, is that grooming tends to be very individualised so we cannot make sweeping generalisations. The predator will work hard to find out what needs the victim has that are not being met, and then set about making promises as to how they will deliver these needs.

HOW TO PROTECT YOUR KIDS FROM ONLINE GROOMING

Beyond being alert and attuned to subtle changes in the demeanour of our children, there are several things we can do to be proactive in protecting our kids from online grooming.

Questioning the questions

Our children will increasingly come into contact with many 'strangers' online and not all of these strangers mean them any harm. In fact, many may become friends. This is why, rather than having a blanket 'stranger danger' approach, we need to teach our kids to be able to better predict the intentions of those we meet online. One way of helping our kids look at the behaviours of others is to question the questions they get asked online.

Whilst some of these questions on their own may be perfectly innocent, when grouped together or asked repeatedly, they should cause us to pause and ask ourselves:

- How do I know this person is actually who they say they are?
- For what purpose does this person need this information about me?
- Why would I be sharing this information and what could be the outcome if they are not in fact who they say they are?

Questions to be alert to include:

- How old are you?
- Are you a boy or a girl?
- Where do you live?
- What are you wearing?
- Are your parents around?
- Want to chat in private?
- Want to move to a different chat site or platform?
- Do your parents check your device?

Managing interactions with people they don't know

Whilst children are young and we do not want them contacted by anyone they don't know, we can:

- Set up filters and settings to keep playing areas private.
- Prevent others from gaining access to them by making all accounts private and turning off new friend requests.
- Speak to our kids about the importance of not giving out personal information online.
- Have young people play in areas where we can hear any banter that may be going on.
- Disallow the use of headphones so we can hear their chats and interactions and listen for inadvertent sharing of information.
- Be sure our kids know how to block and report people.
- Do your research on the places your child is hanging out or wanting to hang out so you know whether they are developmentally appropriate sites or whether you can help set them up in safer ways.

For older kids we can:

- Ensure they are very clear on how to know that someone is who they say they are.

- Never meet someone in real life in a private setting. Always meet in public. Let others know where you are going and preferably bring a friend along.

- Be alert to the requests of others, why they are making those requests and the possible outcomes of sharing information and images online.

Minimising exposure to online predators

We can minimise the chances of our kids being exposed to online predators by:

- Making sure they are playing games that are age-appropriate.

- Always going to the settings button to make the experience as safe as possible.

- Disallowing devices in the bedrooms at night, particularly for primary school-aged children.

- Avoiding having children playing on devices for the same amount of time on the same night every night.

- Ensuring chats don't move from games (like Minecraft and Roblox) to other messaging platforms (like Messenger and WhatsApp).

IMAGE-BASED ABUSE

Whenever we send a naked photo or sexually explicit image of ourselves online it is known as 'sending nudes' or 'sexting'. (Although, please note, these are not usually terms young people use!) Sending nude photos or videos can be done via social media, email, text message or via an online game. And the sending can occur between two people who may or may not be in a relationship, or simply as a way of flirting. Most of the time, this happens with little fallout and the photos/videos are kept relatively private on each person's device.

Sometimes; however, these photos may be shared with a mate, uploaded to a group chat, or added to a sexually explicit website. Whilst they may have been initially sent with consent, the **sharing with others without consent** now renders these images the subject of **image-based abuse**.

'Without consent' also applies when photos are taken without a person's knowledge and shared online. A photo taken up someone's skirt or a video taken in a change room falls in this category. As is a situation like one where my advice was recently sought. A friend took a video of another friend getting changed at a sleepover for a 'laugh'. This video was 'accidentally' airdropped to many other friends and peers at school in amongst a

The most important
thing we need to both
understand and teach
is consent.

group of photos from the evening, resulting in some very distressing fallout.

Image-based abuse also occurs when people are sent nude pictures they don't ask for. These can come from both people who know them (and have them in their contacts) and via unknown accounts on social media. It can also happen when AirDrop is turned on and people take advantage of close proximity to drop nudes onto a person's screen.

UNDERSTANDING CONSENT

When we are talking about sending nude or sexually explicit images or videos, the most important thing we need to both understand and teach is consent. Whilst it can be an offence to have sexually explicit images on our devices, the consequences are certainly amped up when images are sent and shared without consent. Even threatening to share a sexually explicit image of someone can come with a jail term.

At its core, consent is this: when you're engaging in sexual activity (such as sending or receiving nude or sexually explicit images or videos) consent is about communication—clearly telling someone what you intend to do, and receiving their permission or someone clearly telling you what they intend to do, and receiving your permission. It's important to remember that giving consent for one activity, one time, does not mean giving consent for increased or recurring contact of that nature.

Any time we are sending or sharing, or threatening to send or share, sexually explicit images without consent, it comes under the banner of image-based abuse.

This must be reported either to the police or to the appropriate organisations in your country. In Australia, we have the Office of the eSafety Commissioner that has a specific reporting tool for any image-based abuse. They also have a reporting tool for the removal of any sexually explicit image of a person under the age of 18.

Can we safely send nudes?

Whilst this is often seen as a contentious thing to teach young people, it should be noted that sending nude photos can be done in safer ways. For example, if you don't show your face in an image you reduce the likelihood of it being linked to you if that image is leaked.

This harm minimisation approach is one that may well serve our kids' generation better than simply pleading with them to not send nudes. It is also interesting to speak with some young people who are still exploring their sexuality online and via online interactions with others because they actually don't feel ready for the physical intimacy of sex. There is also the reduced likelihood of unwanted pregnancy and STDs when engaging in online encounters!

Of course, this is not going to sit well for everyone. But I do think it is an important aspect to explore when we know there are many people engaging in these behaviours and doing so in risky and dangerous ways.

Other conversations we can have with our kids on this topic are around the fact that:

- Their boyfriend or girlfriend today may not be so in a week or month's time (although of course we all know that this is difficult to concede).

- Once online it is impossible to delete photos or prevent them from being spread. Even photo-sharing apps such as Snapchat which rely on the premise of photos being deleted after a certain amount of time do nothing to stop people screenshotting photos and sharing.

- Revenge porn and bribing people with photos is something that happens regularly and despite now being illegal, it is not something we want our kids involved in (nor do they need an expensive and humiliating court case).

Laws around sending, sharing and receiving sexually explicit images

Different states and countries all have different laws when it comes to the sending and sharing of sexually explicit images. In Victoria, for example, it is still against the law to have nude pictures on your device, but if the ages of the sender and receiver are similar and they were sent with consent, they will no longer find themselves subject to paedophile laws or make their way on to the sex offenders register (as is still the case in some States). Checking individual laws pertaining to your area is the best way to educate young people on their legal rights.

WHAT SHOULD YOU DO IF ...

You are sent a sexually explicit image without consent?

- Delete the photo.
- Block the person if you don't know them.
- Ask that person to refrain from sending you those photos if you do know them.
- If they continue, report that person to the platform, game or social media they are sending the images from.
- If they still persist, in Australia, go to **esafety.gov.au** and report, or go to the police or similar organisation in your country.

A sexually explicit image of yourself is sent online?

- Seek out the support of another trusted person.
- Ask the person who shared the image to take it down.
- If they don't, report that person and the image to the platform, social media or game and ask them to remove it via the reporting tools in the settings.
- In Australia, head to **esafety.gov.au** and report to them the image you would like taken down. If the social network, game or platform has not responded within 48 hours, the eSafety Commissioner can assist in the removal of the images and in some cases take action against the person who shared without consent. Other areas of the world should go to similar organisations or the police.

If someone threatens to share photos to your contacts?

- If someone asks for further pictures or even money in return for not sharing any images of you with your contacts, DO NOT ENGAGE. Report that person and follow up with the eSafety Commissioner or the police if they continue to make threats.

Different states
and countries all
have different laws
when it comes to the
sending and sharing
of sexually explicit
images.

Image-based abuse is a complex and tricky by-product of this uber-connected world. It is a reminder of the magnified and public nature of young people's existence today. Let's keep the conversation going with our young people. Focus not only on their rights to privacy and control of their online images but let's also focus on teaching consent, empathy, trust and respect as being the very building blocks to safe, healthy and positive online experiences.

....
Things to ponder
....

- Do I think my child has the ability to manage online interactions from people they don't know?

- Is there anything going on with their real-world interactions or friendships that would lead them to seek out others online? If so, can they manage to do this in healthy ways?

- How would I react if I found out sexualised images of my child had circulated online? Would I know what steps to take?

- How would I react if my child had circulated or asked for images of others online? Would I know what steps to take?

Conversations to have with your kids

- Do you know how to block someone from your game or social network?

- Do you know how to report someone? What if they continue to harass you?

- What will you do if you are sent pornography, a disturbing video or something that isn't made for young people?

- What clues do you look for to determine someone is who they say they are?

- Are there any questions you could ask a famous person that would prove they are who they say they are? Do you think a famous person would start talking to a young person online in a private chat?

- How can people pretend to be someone else online? How is it different talking to someone online than in real life?

- If you were to meet someone in real life that you met online, what sort of safety precautions would you take?

- Do you know the laws in your area regarding the sending and receiving of sexualised images?

CHAPTER 6

....

DEALING with the dramas
of social media

....

Connecting with people we know, finding new people to connect with, sharing experiences and events, collaborating, chatting and making plans. These have all become the new way of socialising via our social media platforms.

Despite the fact that these social media platforms are created by adults for adults, we also know many young people are spending increasing amounts of time hanging out on them.

And there are definite benefits to doing so:

- They can strengthen their existing relationships with online banter and connection.
- They may find it an easy way to make plans.
- Those isolated or struggling to identify with their immediate peers may 'find their tribe' online.

While many young people have the social, emotional and cognitive maturity to handle the nuances of connecting with others online, there are also many that do not. The maturity, knowledge and skills needed to hang out in these spaces are often lacking in young people making it hard for them to have safe or positive experiences there.

The result can be a whole lot of drama that permeates their online and offline experiences and adds to the already challenging times of growing up, exploring identity, managing hormones, puberty, peer pressure, friendship issues and sexuality.

THE TRAPS OF SOCIAL MEDIA

Here are some of the traps that can have a big impact on us when interacting with others on social media:

1. Comparison

More followers, better holidays, better clothes, better selfies, more money, doing more, being more. Whatever aspect of life we can compare with others, there is no shortage of people online to do this with. For some, this is just a natural part of the online world and it's water off a duck's back. For others, the constant comparison and feeling of not being good enough can be debilitating.

Many social networks have realised this is a problem and have taken steps to negate this reliance on comparison (such as removing the number of likes shown on posts), but the trap of comparison still persists.

2. Exclusion

In my childhood, if there was a party you weren't invited to, you may have been a little upset but soon found yourself engaged with other activities and people over the weekend. Today; however, it is a pretty different story for young people. If there is a party or gathering or sleepover they're not invited to, they can find themselves scrolling through their social media feeds in real-time, witnessing everyone else who is having a great time without them. Seeing picture after picture of people having a good time, live streaming of the event or even people deliberately tagging them in photos amplifies that exclusion.

3. FOMO

Tied closely to these feelings of exclusion are the feelings of FOMO: the Fear Of Missing Out. For some, this means wanting to be constantly connected to their device so they don't miss something. Others need constant reassurance that something is not going on without them.

Whatever aspect of
life we can compare
with others, there
is no shortage of
people online to do
this with.

4. Magnified audience

The problem with the hyperconnected nature of the online world is that when things go wrong, there is a very global, massive and magnified audience that is potentially waiting there to pounce or pile on. So when the wrong picture is uploaded, or we say something thoughtless, or we leave an angry comment on the wrong social influencer's post—the sheer volume of people those things can appear in front of can hugely compound the small feelings of embarrassment, vulnerability and shame we might ordinarily feel about those things.

5. The need to always be 'on'

Many young people have talked to me about feeling that they need to always be 'switched on' and ready to respond; ready to participate in a group chat, answer all those notifications, keep up with the online banter. There are times when they just want to 'chill out' without that threat of missing out or feeling guilty for not constantly responding to friends and peers.

6. Friends vs followers

While it's absolutely possible (and probable) that our kids will meet people online who they will consider to be friends, even if they've never met them before, not all their followers online are likely to be friends. Particularly as they get older and show far less scrutiny on who they will and won't accept into their social media folds. Some kids have well in excess of hundreds or even thousands of followers but are often still only imagining a select group or handful of people on the receiving end of what they post. I've often had young people remark about how they can sometimes be surprised by comments or likes they get from certain people as they weren't necessarily thinking about them when they wrote the post or created the image.

7. Likes vs self-esteem

Social media doesn't affect the self-esteem levels of all kids in the same way. For those already struggling somewhat, or for those who pay a lot of attention to the extrinsic motivators around them, then their experiences on social media can have a considerable impact on their wellbeing. 'Likes' and comments are social currency and become a representation of where they fit in amongst their peers and even society.

TOO MUCH TIME ON SOCIAL MEDIA?

It's not easy to identify how much is 'too much' time spent on social media in a world that is saturated with it. But here are a few signs that social media may not be a good friend to your child's mental health (or yours for that matter):

- Social media disrupts their real-life thoughts and interactions—they are constantly thinking about being online and suffer frequently from FOMO.
- It affects their mood. When they finish scrolling through their feed they're in a worse mood than when they started and their mood is constantly dependent on what happens online.
- Real-life interactions are difficult and being alone is uncomfortable.
- They have no ability to relax or chill out away from screens.
- They find themselves constantly jealous about what others are doing, achieving, seeing, being.
- They relish the misfortune of other.
- They measure their success by the achievements of those they're following online.
- They're addicted to drama and attention, whether good or bad.

Now, of course, many of our children have experienced elements of the above at times, but if these thoughts and behaviours are a constant in their life, then it may be time to look at making some changes.

TIPS FOR MAKING SURE THEIR SOCIAL MEDIA EXPERIENCE IS A GOOD ONE

When comparing online interactions to offline ones, it's clear to see the differences in how our kids communicate, the ways they consume content and the ways they interact with others. By giving them the thinking, the skills and the perspective to understand these nuances, we have a better chance of them avoiding some of that drama, or at least have the skills and knowledge to know how to deal with it in a way that lets them get back to enjoying the positive experiences they can have online.

TIP 1. Think critically about what you post

It sounds obvious that we shouldn't post stuff we don't want others to read. But sometimes the lines get a bit blurred, we forget the audience we are talking to and we get caught up in the moment. Getting our kids to think about what it really means to be a friend, as opposed to what it means to be one of the many amassed followers, can be a great way to start them checking on themselves and being more conscious of all that they share or don't share.

When I'm working with kids I also ask them to think about how comfortable they would be sharing whatever they are posting in front of the whole school assembly, with all the other students, teachers and their parents. Or whether this is something that would probably be best kept within their smaller group of close friends in the playground.

TIP 2. Learn to abort conversations

There will always be people who are wanting to have an argument for argument's sake. They'll get personal with their comments rather than sticking to an issue or the facts at hand.

For this reason, one of the greatest skills we can all acquire today is the ability to know when and how to abort a conversation that isn't going to serve us well. We need to get better at predicting how conversations may play out; at understanding that some people may be more interested in a personal attack than arguing a point of view.

We need to be wary of delving deep into a rabbit hole of back and forth arguments, jibes and comebacks that serve no purpose other than wasting a lot of time, emotional energy and may ultimately be negatively affecting our digital footprint.

There will always
be people who are
wanting to have
an argument for
argument's sake.

Here is an exercise I do with students to get them to think about predicting how a conversation will go and taking the steps to ensure they remain in control. This helps highlight the control they can have over a conversation that isn't having a positive effect on their wellbeing.

> **Lily:** *Why do you always post pictures of your dumb cat? It's so boring!*
>
> **Bella:** *It's better than posting pictures of myself all the time like you do!*
>
> **Lily:** *At least I get heaps more 'likes' on my photos than you do!*
>
> **Bella:** *You don't even know your friends, they are probably creepy old men!*
>
> **Lily:** *You probably only have creepy old cat ladies following you.*
>
> **Bella:** *At least my cat is way better looking than you.*
>
> **Lily:** *Ummm … have you looked at yourself in a mirror lately?*

Once we finish this role play (albeit with a few laughs and gasps in between), the kids are asked to determine who comes across as the mean one in this scenario? Who is not doing their digital footprint any favours? Who is spending a lot of time and energy engaging in an argument they don't seem to be winning, trying to come up with the most powerful responses and generally spending their time online in a really negative way? Most of the time the kids recognise that both Lily and Bella are doing this. Both have equally participated in an online conversation that regardless of who started it, has left them both looking pretty bad and probably had a profound impact on their social and emotional wellbeing.

I then get the kids to discuss other ways they could respond. How do they stay in control? How do they take action to protect themselves, their wellbeing and their digital footprint, despite not having any control over the words and actions of other people? We usually come up with something like this ...

> **Lily:** *Why do you post pictures of your dumb cat? It's so boring!*
>
> **Bella:** *I like my cat. But please feel free to hide my posts for a while if they don't interest you.*
>
> **Lily:** *Well it's obvious everyone else feels the same way.*
>
> **Bella:** *(Ignores, aborts and moves on).*

It is at that point that Bella realises Lily is just up for an argument. It's a fight she's not likely to win nor willing to engage in. She's allowed herself one neutral comment (not nasty or vengeful) and then realised that was enough. She may also have well decided not to respond in the first place and simply ignored or deleted the comment. And that's okay too.

TIP 3. Carefully manage group chats

Group chats can be a great way for a number of people to interact. It can make organising events and outings easy, provide connection and camaraderie, and offer support and friendship in a relatively safe, small and private group.

Like everything online; however, group chats can be used both positively and negatively. Despite the seemingly private and secure nature of group chats, we know that people also sometimes forget that whilst there may be only five people in their chat, there are five sets of parents who are also able to see that chat.

There have also been many times when young people have engaged in nasty behaviour about another person in a group chat, then deliberately invited that person into the chat to see those comments. The deliberate nature of this abuse makes it cyberbullying and something that is unfortunately quite common. I have also had numerous school staff tell me about the group chats that occur late at night, particularly at primary level. The school is asked to manage the behaviours of the people involved in the chat, but more often than not these chats are happening at very late hours of the night. This is another reminder of the role everyone must play in helping to combat negative online experiences.

It's important to get kids to realise that they might be guilty by association, even if they aren't the ones saying the nasty stuff.

Giving young people the skills and the actual words to say should they need to leave a group chat that is getting nasty is also a skill in itself. Coming up with actual words to say, for example, 'Sorry guys, this is getting pretty nasty, I'm outta here' or just 'Sorry guys, gotta go' are some of the examples kids have given me. Simply leaving the chat is okay too.

TIP 4. Learn to respond rather than react

There are going to be times when people make us mad online. Times when their points of view make them less than amiable; when their comments are said to get a rise out of others; when we just can't understand why people will do and say the things they do online. Learning to take the time to respond to other people rather than simply react is a useful skill for us all.

Kids have given me all sorts of ideas to have as their response plan for when things don't go well online.

Things such as:

- Turning off for a while, playing a different game, changing servers or seeking out something positive online.

- Talking it out with people in real life if it is a friend or peer that has upset them online.

- Doing something active to have some time out. Kick a ball, shoot some hoops, walk the dog.

- Doing something to calm themselves, such as reading a book, drawing, watching some TV.

- Typing out a response to someone but not hitting 'send'.

- Sleeping on it. Always wait until the next day if you think you may respond in a way that you could possibly regret. We always feel differently about situations after we've had time to process. More often than not we will come to the conclusion that it just isn't worth the effort or the emotional energy.

TIP 5. Learn to shrug

On a recent visit to the gym, one of the exercises we were doing was working the trapezius muscle. When we finished, the instructor reminded us that this was the muscles we use to shrug. To shrug our shoulders and get on with life. Really useful muscles. And I have to

Like everything online, group chats can be used both positively and negatively.

agree. Today more than ever we need to work on these muscles that allow us to shrug.

The online world opens us up to so many people. So many opinions. So many beliefs. So many different life experiences. So many judgements. So many points of view. So many people with ulterior motives. So many nasty, vitriolic, jealous, bitter, and downright crazy people.

There are times we need to respond to these people, to call out the bad behaviours. Times we need to stick up for a mate or even a stranger. Times we should assert our right to an opinion without being belittled, judged or harassed. There are times when we need to use the tools at our disposal to block, delete and report.

But there are also times when we need to just shrug. For our own wellbeing it can be a really useful skill. It helps us leave some of the bitterness and anger behind. I use it now for those times I read something that makes me think, 'What in the world's name are they thinking?' or 'How could people ever come to that conclusion?' or 'Man I wish they would just stop typing or tweeting or posting'.

At the end of the day, it is difficult to change people online. We can try and enlighten them and we can certainly call out the deplorable behaviour when it is warranted. But there is a certain amount of stuff that happens that just requires a good shrug. And those are times we need to encourage our kids to lift up their shoulders, take a deep breath, drop their shoulders, exhale and say to themselves: 'Not my problem ... not today ... I'm moving on.'

TIP 6. Apply empathy online

The online world thus becomes an easy place to lay judgement, especially if we couple that with the protection of hiding behind a keyboard or communicating anonymously.

Which is why being able to understand and share the feelings of someone else is certainly becoming a crucial skill for our children to foster today.

To help build kids' empathy we need to encourage them to know what it feels like to walk in someone else's shoes. To examine the biases they may already hold due to their own situations and circumstances and to look at how this may affect the way they see the world as opposed to the beliefs and values of other people.

We can encourage our kids to ask questions. To learn about others. To be curious about the world around them. When we have a developed sense of empathy we are also able to look out for others around us, be an upstander and assert everyone's right to be treated with respect.

Things to ponder

- How much value does my child place on the validation they get (or not) from social media?
- Are they showing signs that their online experiences are having a negative impact on their wellbeing?
- Do they have plenty of other pursuits, role models and achievements outside their online world?
- Are they getting plenty of opportunities to thrive in the real world?
- Are they the type of child to take things to heart, or are they pretty resilient when it comes to their understanding of how online interactions play out?

Conversations to have with your kids

- Can you differentiate between a friend and a follower? What sorts of things would you share with a friend that you wouldn't with your followers?
- How does it make you feel when you see other people getting lots of likes, friends and followers or sharing their seemingly perfect life?

- What are some things you could do if you knew you weren't invited to a party and people were going to be posting and sharing pictures of that party?

- When should you move a conversation with a friend offline? What can be the consequences of having sensitive conversations online?

- Do you know when and how to abort a conversation that isn't going to end well?

- What are some phrases that may help you leave a conversation?

- What are your boundaries around blocking people? When would you report someone?

- Why is it difficult to change someone's mind in an online conversation?

- What would you do in a group chat if things got nasty or deliberately excluded someone?

- What are some of the different situations that people may be going through that may determine how they react online?

- How can people's past experiences, values or circumstances influence how they think and behave and what they believe?

- What are some ways you could help in your community? What interests, groups, clubs are you involved in that could use your skills to ensure you are building your self worth from a variety of means?

CHAPTER 7

··

BUILDING the knowledge to deal with cyberbullying

··

Cyberbullying is certainly one of the greatest downsides to a world that relies on interaction and connections in order to learn, inform, work and socialise within online platforms. When bullying is occurring in the place where one is spending much of their time, the effects can range from frustration, sadness and anxiety to anger, depression and even suicide.

Whilst there are many factors that may determine the level and effect bullying behaviours have on different people and their ability to respond to these behaviours, there are certainly ways we can help minimise those effects and give our kids the skills and understanding to face cyberbullying.

WHAT DOES CYBERBULLYING LOOK LIKE?

In essence, it can be described as bullying that occurs via electronic or digital means. We have laws established to protect those being cyberbullied, and we need our kids to know and understand these behaviours as well as the process to follow should they need to deal with cyberbullying either themselves or for someone else.

The following behaviours can all come under the banner of cyberbullying when they include the intent to cause harm or embarrassment, when they involve a power imbalance and when they happen repeatedly, despite a request for the behaviour to stop:

- The sending of threatening or harassing text, email or chat messages either privately, publicly or as a group chat.
- Impersonating another person, either by hacking into an account or creating an account with the intent to come across as someone else.
- Abusing another player in an online game.
- The uploading and sharing of images or videos without consent in order to hurt or embarrass.
- Stalking or repeatedly making contact with someone when they have asked you to stop or taken steps to block or report.

It's important young people know that while we throw the word bullying around quite readily these days, there is a difference between bullying that occurs online, and generally mean and nasty stuff that may also be experienced. That mean and nasty behaviour is often labelled as bullying but it is actually more people failing to think things through and being bitchy, narcissistic, jealous or just thriving on the drama.

Why do we need to differentiate? Because while all mean behaviour is hurtful, bullying needs to be dealt with differently.

We need to be careful we don't become nonchalant to the impact and effect of bullying and ensure we follow the right processes to stop bullying behaviour in its tracks.

WHAT ARE THE SIGNS OF A CHILD BEING CYBERBULLIED?

This can be pretty tricky to ascertain as kids are very good at covering up cyberbullying. We know this because the statistics repeatedly tell us the disparity between the number of young people being bullied and those sharing those incidents with an adult. But some of the warning signs that may ensure you investigate further are:

Being mean or nasty online is not the same as cyberbullying. They are two different things and they need to be dealt with differently.

- being secretive about their time on devices
- being emotionally withdrawn
- refusing to discuss online activities
- a lack of motivation to do the things they once enjoyed (sports, extracurricular activities, hanging with friends etc)
- mood changes after being on a device or gaming
- a refusal to go to school or other social outings.

WHAT TO DO IF YOUR CHILD IS CYBERBULLIED

It is important young people feel safe and supported when cyberbullying has occurred. The end result must be that the bullying stops. The child must feel that this is the goal being worked towards and that their life will not be made more difficult as a result of any action taken.

Parents and children should try to mutually agree on a plan of action. Whilst this can be a highly emotional and stressful time, parents must try to remain rational and logical so as not to make the situation worse.

While different situations and circumstances will call for different paths of action, the following procedures may be included:

- Contacting your child's school to organise a meeting (if the cyberbullying is coming from another student).

- Contacting social media or gaming platforms to have the offending material removed. (In Australia, we have the Office of the eSafety Commissioner to report and follow the process to remove material and follow up if necessary.)

- Contacting the police if bullying is of a threatening nature and the child feels unsafe, or if a crime has been committed, ie stalking, blackmail, sexual exploitation etc.

- Keeping records and taking screenshots of bullying incidents if they are escalating.

It's important that, as a parent, you do not personally approach the child perpetrating the behaviour.

WHAT IF YOUR CHILD IS CYBERBULLYING?

Sometimes kids lack empathy, act out their own pain in ways that hurt others or get wrapped up in the 'gang mentality' of copying and following the negative behaviours of others. It's important to understand where your child's bullying is coming from in order to address those behaviours.

There may also need to be some consequences such as the times the child is allowed access online, removing access at nighttime and discussing together why changes need to be made to their online use in order to reflect the behaviours you expect. It's important your child understands how their behaviour is harmful to both the child being bullied and themselves.

Just as it is difficult to determine if your child is being cyberbullied, it can be equally, if not more difficult to know if your child is cyberbullying others. Some signs to look out for may be:

- wanting to access the internet at all hours, including late at night
- quickly switching between screens when you walk in the room
- having multiple accounts for the one network
- gets moody or upset if they don't have access to their device.

If you have been approached by the school or other parents, it is important to listen to those accusations and discuss in a calm manner to try and ascertain the truth, rather than blindly denying such accusations.

WHOSE RESPONSIBILITY IS IT TO DEAL WITH CYBERBULLYING?

It's *everyone's* responsibility.

Whilst schools need the help of parents, parents also need the help of schools.

We also need the help of government organisations to regulate, put pressure on the designers of the social networks, and maintain pressure on the big tech companies to do the right things by their users.

And of course, we need society as a whole to look out for each other and put boundaries around behaviours that won't be tolerated. It can be difficult as parents often feel out of their depth in dealing with an environment they are not comfortable or entirely familiar with. Law enforcement and schools are also not always sure of their role and where their responsibility extends. And so with still a lot of uncertainty in this space, we must continue to seek out those that can help support young people during these times as well as provide the education to know the options that are there for them to put an end to cyberbullying.

HOW TO PREVENT CYBERBULLYING

It is obviously very difficult to control how other people behave. We have little say in the words others use or the ways they abuse the technology to inflict harm on others. But there are some things we can do to minimise the occurrence and the impact, and take steps to prevent the exposure of young people to cyberbullying behaviours.

- Be clear about the types of behaviours that are not to be tolerated and of course those behaviours that they are not to engage in themselves.

- Develop resilience to ignore the minor name-calling, or mean and nasty behaviours so these situations do not escalate to bullying.

- Make sure children know how to delete people, block people and report on every single game and app they play.

- Go through the account privacy settings regularly to ensure they are creating the safest environment for themselves to play in.

- Ensure they have a trusted relationship with another adult and discuss the importance of needing help when things go wrong online.

- Remain relevant to your child's world by understanding how the technology works, by talking to them about their experiences and by

It's not just the
school's or the parents'
responsibility to deal
with cyberbullying,
it's **everyone's**
responsibility.

avoiding making technology 'the bad guy'. We want kids to come to us should things go wrong online, without the threat of having all of their technology access shut down or taken away.

ENCOURAGING BYSTANDERS TO BE UPSTANDERS

There are many times where young people will witness cyberbullying but feel reluctant to get involved. They either fear the repercussions or don't feel they have the skills or knowledge to support people in these circumstances.

Unfortunately; however, by doing nothing we are accepting the behaviours and even passively encouraging them.

By taking an active role and upstanding, a person can have a great impact on stopping the bullying.

- They could simply approach the target of the bullying in real life and help and encourage them to get some help.

- They may help them block or report people.

- They may respond online to the negative comments with an encouraging or positive comment to the target or even a comment to the perpetrator to stop their behaviour.
- They may also save the digital evidence if this is something they think is likely to escalate.

Obviously the level of upstanding will depend on a person's confidence and resilience. It may also be easier done when a few friends can join together and feel the power in numbers.

....

Things to ponder

....

- Would I be able to tell if my child was being cyberbullied?
- Would I know if my child was cyberbullying another?
- Does my child have times when they are away from the screens to have a mental break from their online interactions?
- Would I know what to do if I discovered my child was involved in a cyberbullying incident?

Conversations to have with your kids

- What would you do if you could see that a friend or peer was being bullied online?

- Why is it so hurtful to be cyberbullied? How does it differ from the words we have in real life?

- Whose responsibility is it to look after people online? What roles should the social networks and gaming platforms have? What involvement should schools have? When should parents be involved?

- Would you be comfortable in sticking up for someone who was being bullied?

- In what ways can you help others if they are being cyberbullied?

- Do you have someone you can turn to if you were experiencing bullying?

- Do you feel supported by friends, parents, teachers or the school?

CHAPTER 8

....

SEEING the good in the online world

....

It's easy to get so caught up in the negative experiences our kids might have online, that we miss the many wonderful benefits: potential for greater connection, increased access to information, social change and awareness, creativity, collaboration and of course convenience and greater work flexibility.

The fact we're all so immersed in the online world suggests there must actually be much to love about this new way of learning, interacting, connecting, sharing, informing, entertaining and let's face it … filling in time.

Ultimately, the online world isn't going anywhere fast so here are some thoughts about how we can take advantage of all of the opportunities it presents.

IT PRESENTS OPPORTUNITIES FOR SOCIAL GOOD

One of my favourite things about the online world is the way it gives our kids a heightened sense of social awareness and is helping them become active citizens in ways that help implement change and raise awareness of issues.

Some 8-year-old daughters of a friend had learnt about endangered species at school and wanted to do something active to help make a difference. They were not overly outgoing or extroverted but had found an issue they were passionate about. They decided they wanted to create a GoFundMe page to raise money for koalas. Each day they would share drawings of koalas they created and in return would ask for small donations from friends and family to help their cause. The result was not only the raising of some funds for their cause but also an awareness for these girls that they can do positive things in the world despite little resources or finances of their own.

When we are helping others we are also helping to feel worthwhile and thus helping to build important feelings of self-esteem. Whilst these girls may grow up to witness a whole lot of bad stuff online, the hope also is that they have already witnessed the ways it can be used in positive ways and it is more likely they will continue to focus on those, rather than seek out the negative elements.

IT OFFERS EMOTIONAL FREEDOM— PARTICULARLY TO BOYS

I used to love watching the emotion I would see from boys and men on a sporting field as they hugged fellow players, cried in happiness and sadness and kissed their teammates. It always proved to me that they crave not only the outpouring of this emotion but the connection with others in a way that didn't call them out as 'sissy'.

It's been surprising for me to discover the role social media is playing in breaking down the traditional notion of boys being emotionally stoic and unable to show vulnerable emotion for fear of being called out as 'less manly'.

I recently observed the social media feeds of my teenage son and was pleasantly surprised at the love these friends have for each other. There were kisses, and love heart emojis amongst all the 'love you bro's'.

Now, of course, it is easier to be that way online than in real life and some of it may certainly be 'tongue in cheek'. But it certainly shows that we all have a need for connection and outward emotion, and it's possible social media will help to make this okay and even make it the norm.

When we are
helping others we
are also helping to
feel worthwhile and
thus helping to build
important feelings
of self-esteem.

IT GIVES KIDS THE CHANCE TO BE SEEN AND HEARD

We all know people tend to be braver online with their words than they are in real life. And we talk often about the negative impact of the keyboard warriors hurling their abuse and personal attacks while they remain tucked safely behind the screen.

There is a positive side to this however. For those young people who are shy, introverted, and maybe not given a platform before, the online world is a place for them to have a voice and feel heard. They can publicly present themselves in a way they may not otherwise be able to or inclined to do, in real life. It's no surprise that when you walk into a room full of bloggers or social media influencers, a large majority are usually shy and far more socially anxious in real life, whilst their online spaces give them a place to more confidently share their voice.

IT ALLOWS KIDS TO TAP INTO THEIR CREATIVITY

We often hear the cries of kids being 'dumbed down' and turning into zombies as they stare at their phones, but there can be an awful lot of creativity going on with those swipes. One only has to see some of the amazing cities, buildings and stadiums young people create using tools such as Minecraft, as well as the music videos, podcasts, photos and songs that can be created by the many apps that allow an enormous amount of creative freedom and expression.

Young people are constantly taking photos, filming videos and finding content to share and comment on. Discovering new content and modifying and critically evaluating it, both as a representation of what they believe and as a way to express themselves and their ideas and beliefs, is fast becoming the norm.

IT OFFERS THE GIFT OF ACCESS

Once again, we have to acknowledge that having access to multitudes of information and content is not always a good thing. But if we also look at this as a wonderful gift of having access to the world in ways that can help educate, work, grow, connect and collaborate, then it certainly has the ability to change the lives of so many for the better.

The online world allows us to do things like:

- getting in touch with our favourite authors and invite them into the classroom via a Skype call
- seeking out real-time footage of people and places far and wide, to see firsthand the landscapes, buildings and animals in action

- watching concerts and speeches live
- working from home in a way that allows for greater flexibility of our lifestyles
- contacting friends and family anywhere, at almost any time
- making plans that may have to change at any time knowing that we can easily make those changes
- calling our kids to make sure they arrived somewhere safely
- getting our groceries delivered if we can't get out of the house or make it to the shops.

There is certainly much to appreciate about how technology has changed our lives for the better. So much so, we must continue to seek out those positive ways and be intentional with our use, so the ledger is always in favour of what's being added to our lives rather than what is being taken away.

20 WAYS TO USE THE ONLINE WORLD IN A POSITIVE WAY

1. Write a list of historical moments you would like to know more about—events you never learnt about in school but would like a little more understanding of. Next time you are bored, pop one in a Google search and see what you discover.

2. Grab a series of photos—maybe from a recent holiday, or any event—put them in a slideshow, add some music and create a short video masterpiece.

3. Interview your kids using the video feature on your phone. Ask them any number of random questions and you have a priceless keepsake.

4. Get your kids to interview you. Ask them to think of some questions, maybe about your childhood, your early memories of them as a child. What a great keepsake for them too.

5. Write something. Get out a Notes app or Google Docs and just write: a journal entry, a poem, that book you wanted to start.

6. Send a message, text or email to someone to tell them you appreciate them or admire something they have achieved.

7. Search a recipe of something you've never cooked and give it a whirl.

8. If you've never done meditation, search for an app and find your zen.

9. Think of a new skill you would like to learn and see if you can get some pointers online.

10. Download a reading app, grab a book online and always have something on the go you can reach for in those downtimes.

11. Search a podcast, maybe a subject area you don't know a lot about, pop the headphones in and make those mundane chores a little more bearable.

12. Go through your emails and unsubscribe to any you haven't opened recently.

13. Delete any apps on your phone you haven't used in the last few months.

14. Make a playlist of your favourite songs, or songs from different eras or different moods.

15. Use the recording feature to record messages, thoughts or ideas with your voice for those moments you can't type or write.

16. Read a bookmarked article or saved video. We are not always in the headspace to read articles we are interested in at the time we are scrolling, but having them saved somewhere for easy access will ensure they don't get forgotten.

17. Play a game of Words with Friends, chess, or any game that gets those brain cells ticking over.

18. Is there a language you've always wanted to learn? Maybe you see some exotic travel destination in your future where knowing a few phrases could be of help. There are plenty of apps for that.

There is certainly
much to appreciate
about how technology
has changed our lives
for the better.

19. Find a quick workout to get moving even if only for 10 minutes. Maybe you don't want to start doing burpees or squats whilst you're waiting in the supermarket queue, but if you have space and a few minutes, there are plenty of online workouts to keep you active.

20. Finally, this one requires leaving the phone at home (or keeping it in the back pocket if you want to track your distance travelled): head out for a big walk (or even a little one) and breathe in the fresh air. Explore the world around you, take note of your senses, what can you see, feel and hear that you usually wouldn't?

....

Things to ponder

....

- Could there be ways of using social media that may be benefitting my child?

- Could we be seeking out positive experiences together online?

- Am I subconsciously focusing on the bad things that happen online and the content I don't want them to see, rather than balancing that with positive talk about what is out there and what is possible?

Conversations to have with your kids

- Who are the people online that you have seen make a positive difference to the world?

- How have people managed to use social media for good?

- Have you witnessed positive change online via social networks globally or from your peers?

- In what other ways could we use social media to create positive outcomes?

- How can you ensure the content you create (pictures, writing, videos, podcasts etc) will have a positive impact on other people's online experiences?

CHAPTER 9

....

MANAGING screen time effectively

....

Managing screen time is less of a technology problem that needs to be managed and more of an overall attention and intention issue. Why? Because the people who create the technology and systems that are keeping us so occupied are doing so with the goal to keep us online longer. They want us to use their products. They have the knowledge and research to know what our brains respond to. And thus they engineer things to make it as difficult as possible for us to push back against.

Given that effectively managing screen time can be difficult for adults, it is surely going to be something kids need some help with.

HOW MUCH SCREEN TIME IS TOO MUCH?

This question is asked by parents all the time as they struggle to feel in control of the amount of time their child uses screens and technology. And the truth is, there is no easy answer. In fact, I usually answer this question with three more of my own.

Q1. What is your child doing on the screens?

- Are they consuming a copious amount of irrelevant, inappropriate content? Or are they researching, learning and developing ideas and thinking?

- Are they researching how to make a paper aeroplane to fly with their brother? Or are they watching something violent? (Two vastly different ways to spend 30 minutes on YouTube.)

- Are they creating, making and producing their own content or are they merely consuming? Are they watching some guy unbox toys for hours on end or are they creating a song on GarageBand or making a movie on iMovie?

- Are they playing a couple of quick video games after school to de-stress or have a social chat with their mates, or are they playing games that are inappropriate in nature, content and themes and leave them feeling aggressive, moody and unwilling to participate in other activities?

- Are they sharing and consuming inspiring and positive media or are they feeding their insecurities and damaging their sense of self-worth?

- Are they showing responsibility, leadership, empathy or kindness with the content they share, or are they disrespecting themselves or others?

- Are they left alone for hours on their own, shut up in a room, or are parents sitting, engaging, pointing out, asking questions, inferring outcomes and connecting and bonding with their child together?

It is, of course, okay for kids to scroll through the social media feeds of their friends and to watch YouTube videos that don't always have an educational element. It is okay for them to use technology to relax and be entertained. But we do want to emphasise to them that for the majority of their time online, the way they are using screens should be having a positive effect on their lives and wellbeing.

Q2. What effect is the screen time having on your child?

- Are they engaging in positive interactions, having a laugh with mates and maintaining and developing positive friendships and connections? Or are they experiencing drama, bullying others or being bullied themselves?

For the majority
of their time online,
our kids' screen
use should have
a positive effect
on their lives and
wellbeing.

- Are they feeling happy when they turn off the screens or are they anxious, depressed or aggressive?

- Are they enjoying banter with friends and peers or are they feeling the pressure of trying to keep up and stay connected?

- Are they struggling to stand up for someone and avoid peer pressure or are they taking a stand for those who are unable?

- Is their self-esteem constantly being challenged? Or are they able to shrug off the comparisons? Are they okay to move on and remain confident in themselves and their place in this world?

- Is the normally introverted shy child finding a voice online for a cause they are passionate about when they usually wouldn't have the confidence?

Experiences online are not always going to be rosy, fun and full of positivity. But for the most part, we want to look at how we can help kids seek out the experiences and people that will help them find those moments and to give them the knowledge, skills and understanding to avoid those negative effects and minimise the harm they can bring.

Q3. What are they missing out on?

- Are they able to happily come to the dinner table, get plenty of sleep at night, and still do their chores and keep up with homework? Or are they having a tantrum every time they are told to put away the device?

- Are they still engaging with the friends and extracurricular activities they have always enjoyed or are they becoming reclusive and unengaged?

- Are they taking time to walk the dog after school, hang out with friends or siblings or are they staying inside their room from the moment they get home until they are called for dinner?

- Are they having opportunities to reflect, to ponder things, to chill out, without feeling 'socially switched on' 24/7?

Devices are certainly here to stay for the foreseeable future so we need to get smarter about how we all approach our screen time experiences. Looking at the cognitive, social and emotional effects, both positive and negative, as well as looking at the particular needs and circumstances of an individual child, will go a long way to getting the balance right and ensuring they remain in control of their screen time experiences.

HOW TO KNOW IF *YOUR* CHILD IS HAVING TOO MUCH SCREEN TIME

So you've asked yourself the three questions above but you're still not sure whether your child is getting 'too much' screen time or not. Here are two key indicators that they might be tipping too far in the wrong direction.

1. They are exhibiting obsessive behaviours

There is no doubt there is a small percentage of the population whose online behaviours have become obsessive and may in some instances be called addictive.

If your child is in 'red flag' territory where they are exhibiting obsessive behaviours but they haven't tipped over into addiction, then you manage things by slowly cutting back the time they're spending on screens (rather than going cold turkey).

If a child is becoming violent and aggressive; however, and missing out on vital hours of sleep or refusing to go to school or participate in other activities, then these issues may certainly need to be dealt with by seeking professional help. In situations such as this, there are also likely to be other areas of concern that go beyond the lure of the games and technology that would likely need to be addressed.

2. They are having trouble fitting in 'all the things'

As we wrestle with all the things that are there vying for our attention, it becomes imperative that we help our kids maintain some control over that pull. I ask parents to remind their kids that we are not putting boundaries around their device use because we want to be mean and controlling. Rather, it's because we want them to have the time to fit all the things they need.

- Time to be active and to exercise.
- Time to play.
- Time to connect with others in real life.
- Time to work.
- Time to eat.
- Time to sleep.
- Time to let our mind wander.

It's these moments of mind-wandering that allow us all to think more creatively, to become curious and to slow down a little without feeling like we are constantly filling our minds and every moment with stuff. If our kids have no space in there for 'boredom' and mind-wandering, then there's a good chance they're spending too much time on screens.

THE MYTH OF MULTITASKING

One of the big challenges of the digital age is the belief that we can multitask—that managing many tasks at once allows us to get more done faster, which should, in theory, free up more time.

But not many people seem to be less busy these days! So something isn't working.

Just because we can scroll, tweet, like, comment, share, play a round of Words with Friends, crush some candy and answer an email whilst cooking, vacuuming, walking, driving, talking, lunching or partaking in a myriad of other tasks doesn't mean we should.

Because there is no such thing as multitasking. What we're actually doing is task switching. And every time we take our brain attention away from one task and move it, even briefly, to another, it takes away the effectiveness of both tasks. Our brain needs to regroup every time we change focus and thus we lose time and efficiency.

While your child might think they can scroll that feed, respond to a Snapchat sent, listen to a

If kids have no
space for boredom
and mind-wandering,
then there's a good
chance they're
spending too much
time on screens.

podcast, buy that dress from the online store all while learning a new skill, idea or concept, the reality is vastly different:

- Tasks take longer due to this changing of focus. It is estimated that it can take up to five minutes to get back to a task after leaving it to answer an email or respond to a text.
- We suffer from mental fatigue more quickly and thus are more likely to make errors. Studies have found, unsurprisingly, that those given three tasks made three times as many mistakes as those given two (i.e. the more tasks, the more mistakes).
- Memory is impaired, resulting from reduced attention span, learning and performance.

HOW TO BE MORE INTENTIONAL ABOUT THE TIME SPENT ON SCREENS

Here are some thoughts and guidelines around managing screen time in an intentional fashion (rather than a heavily rule-driven one).

1. Set screen time limits

I always advocate that time limits can be useful for younger kids to set them on a path to being able to regulate their time and spend it in ways that recognise there are always be many other needs that need to be met.

- Start young with time limits so kids know that the devices are there for just a small part of their day. During the toddler and preschool years, their development still requires so many other activities that don't require a screen.

- Help them understand the concept that screens are just one element of their play and learning by providing other activities for them to go on with once they have had some time with a screen. This helps them recognise that they are not being punished by having the devices taken away, they just have other activities that they can easily transition to.

- Don't frame the technology as a forbidden fruit as such, but keep it as something that is a 'sometimes' tool. A bit like the cakes and biscuits which are generally going to be okay for your child, as long as they are getting plenty of the fruit and vegetables.

- Recognise that time limits are going to be much harder and likely to become redundant once a child hits school age and older. When they are using devices for homework and greater connection with friends and the devices become more and more a part of their day, that's when we want to be teaching them the skills to use screens with intention. We can still have boundaries around certain times they use the devices, i.e., not at the dinner table or late at night, but we are wanting them to start to play a bigger role in how they manage those devices in ways that give them some autonomy to do that themselves. This is obviously easier with some kids than with others.

2. Differentiate between intentional use and mindless use

It is certainly a tricky scenario we have set up for ourselves when the work, learning and studying that needs to be done, must also be done whilst using these very devices that provide so much distraction. I'm often hearing parents lament that they have no idea whether their child is actually doing the homework they say they are doing, or whether they are chatting to friends, playing games or watching NBA playoffs on YouTube. Here are some questions we might want our kids to ask themselves:

Are you mindlessly scrolling?

Are you just scrolling the feeds of people you don't really have a connection to? Businesses you will never buy from? Celebrities you will never relate to? Status updates of stuff you don't really need to see on a daily basis? Are you just scrolling on by hoping to be awakened by something that catches our attention for longer than a millisecond?

Who are you following and why?

Are the people you follow providing you with support, friendship and connection? Are they teaching you, motivating you, challenging you or inspiring you? Are they people you can help or support? If so, then the time you spend engaging with them is likely to be worth that investment. If however you have no real connection, they say things that upset you, they erode your sense of self-esteem, they bring down your mood, they make you feel less than worthy, then they are not a good investment. Cull them now and tidy up your feeds.

What are you consuming?

Is the media you're reading or watching balanced and truthful? Should you be seeking a wider variety of news or opinion? Are you reading the same sort of things over and over? Would it be worthwhile to be a little more intentional about how you receive and form your view of the world?

What exactly are you spending your time on?

Surfing the net may certainly be a very worthwhile way to spend your day. You may be researching, learning a new language, collating home videos, playing a game that relaxes you and relieves stress. You may be entertained in ways that give you enjoyment and add positivity to your day. But maybe there are games to play that are more creative or challenging? Maybe watching some dude unbox toys is not the most productive use of your time. Maybe there is a better way to spend your time than clicking through Facebook posts to determine which member of the Royal family you most look like, or how many children is the perfect number for you (as a mother to five boys it is rather unsettling to discover that two was indeed a perfect number for me!).

If we can be confident our kids are paying attention to how they are using their devices and that they are aware of the effects those experiences are having on them, then we can care less about addictions, time-wasting and overuse. We can also care less about bullying, comparison, judgment and exclusion because they will already be addressing these people and situations as unworthy recipients of their time.

3. Getting help from the technology itself

In order to focus on certain tasks at certain times, we may need to look at other strategies to help our kids get back on track. In order to filter out the noise so we can concentrate on certain important tasks, we may ironically need the help of the technology on offer.

Start young with
time limits so kids
know that the devices
are there for just a
small part of
their day.

- There are apps that help us manage our time and count down study and work periods in order to provide that one-dimensional focus. (See the resource page of my website for a list of these.)

- There are filtering systems that also work with your WiFi connection or with your device itself to turn off certain apps that are going to be distracting at certain times. That way your kids won't be tempted to respond to notifications, or get stuck scrolling that feed.

- We can all turn off the notifications and big red circles that alert us someone else is vying for our attention. Even the sound or the sight of a notification is enough to distract us, even if we don't open and respond to it.

- We can make our devices less appealing by setting them to greyscale via the settings of the device. The less colourful those apps are, the less appealing they are to the brain.

- We can 'hide' those apps that are the greatest culprits in snatching our attention by moving them further away from the home page or hiding them in folders, so they are not so easily clickable.

- Close down the tabs. If you're working on something important, close down all the other tabs to remove the lure of being one click away from a distraction rabbit hole.

Things to ponder

- What is the current role screens play in my child's life?
- What messages am I sending around screen time behaviours and managing my time?
- Is my child able to, for the most part, fit in all the things they need to happen in their day?
- Do I feel in a position to help my child make changes that will help them find greater balance with their time management?
- Do I feel there are areas of my child's life that are lacking or beginning to slide?
- Am I paying attention to any red flags or sudden changes in moods and behaviours?

Conversations to have with your kids

- Do you know why it is important to have good habits around our time on screens and our attention to devices?
- Do you feel there are areas of your life not given the attention they deserve?

- Do you feel overwhelmed by the constant need to check your device, maintain online interactions or group chats?

- Do you find yourself easily distracted and notice seemingly small tasks take much longer to complete?

- What are some things you can do to make sure you are better able to achieve balance and be more intentional with the way you use your device?

- Do you see real benefit with the people you follow, the information served up to you, the connections you engage with and the sorts of online pursuits you spend your time on? Could you be more intentional with the way you spend your precious time and energy?

CHAPTER 10

··

GAMING in a healthy way

··

Video games tend to get a bad rap from media, parents and society as a whole as the world laments the impact they've had on a nostalgic world of books, board games and outside play.

Yes, they can while away many hours from a child's day, promote violent play and misogynistic themes and prevent children from getting the exercise and sleep they need.

But they are also a valid form of entertainment, storytelling, pastime, social platform and sometimes even a stress reliever that can be a perfectly healthy addition to our children's lives.

Like all modern-day developments, we should get active and empowered about the role these relatively new toys will play. Rather than cower in a world of anxiety and fear, constantly clicking on the alarmist headlines, let's instead take the reins and choose to work with our kids and the technology to ensure it can be a positive addition to their lives.

THE POSITIVE ASPECTS OF GAMING

I first need to make it clear that I would never advocate for a child to play video games non-stop at the expense of their wellbeing. It goes without saying that they should not be playing games so much that they don't get any homework done, or that they skip meals or sleep or stop hanging out with friends or doing activities they always did. I am also not advocating for young children to play inappropriate and violent games that are sending all sorts of crazy messages about violence, gender roles, breaking the law etc.

There are; however, many, many video games out there that are actually great for your child as well as being something they simply enjoy doing. And there has been a significant increase in research in this area. The findings of researchers such as Daphne Bavelier and Jane McGonigal dismiss the notion of gaming as being mindless and time-wasting, but rather espouse the benefits of gaming to actually ignite positive change to social, emotional, physical and cognitive development.

If your child loves playing games, instead of spending all your energy worrying about how you can stop them from playing, remember that there are some really good reasons why you should continue to let them play.

1. Gaming provides a sense of achievement

Going through different levels, accomplishing tasks, gaining access to new worlds or environments and creating and making things, allows them to feel the excitement and satisfaction of achievement. For children who may struggle to attain a certain level of success in other more 'popular' arenas, the positive benefits of conquering a game or level can never be underestimated for its ability to boost confidence and create a positive sense of self.

2. Gaming increases coordination and tracking skills

The physical benefits of game playing also refer to improvements in spatial awareness, hand-eye coordination and attention to detail, not to mention the physical benefits of movement from exercise games such as Wii. Higher spatial resolution in visual processing has also been seen to be transferable to spatial tasks outside the game. Many careers now use gaming as part of their training to simulate situations and build on these skills.

Conquering a game
or level can boost
confidence and
create a positive
sense of self.

3. Games provide a sense of belonging

For many children, video games give them a sense of belonging they may not get to experience in other areas of their lives. Not all kids get to feel the sense of community from their peers, they may not enjoy sports and being part of a team, they may not have any other avenue of feeling connected. Many who have become involved in the world of gaming speak of the sense of being part of a community. With over 70% of game playing involving collaboration or competition this also emphasises the interactive nature of video games as opposed to the more passive nature of other screen time activities. Collaborative games can also require leadership and decision making skills as we can see in group games such as Minecraft. Even those that watch other players without even playing, feel a sense of being part of something. As long as the connections remain positive, then this can only be a good thing.

4. Gaming is good for stress release

When kids get home from school sometimes they need time to 'switch off'. Having to participate, to be 'on', be present and interacting with others all day can be emotionally taxing on many kids. Often that is the reason we don't get a lot of conversation out of them when they first walk in the door. They need time to unwind. Video games have been reported to have huge benefits for those needing to simply 'chill out' for a while and do their own thing without the demands of others. It can also be a safe environment to manage negative emotions. Once again as long as these are not replacing all other avenues of downtime and relaxation, then gaming can be one way to negate the stresses of everyday life.

5. Gaming develops persistence and resilience

Persistence and overcoming obstacles is one of the most valuable skills we can teach our kids. Many video games require you to experiment with different ways to do things. They require you to change tactics, be creative in your thinking and strategy and come up with new ways to solve problems. I can think of numerous careers where these skills are highly beneficial and certainly persistence, an ability to change and adapt and to think outside the box are the greatest assets to a resilient mindset.

6. Gaming is good for cognitive thinking

Gaming is not always about shooting people, or racing cars. And even in these games as well as the many other types of games kids play, there is some pretty high order thinking that is required to conquer challenges, solve puzzles and advance to other levels.

7. Gaming is good for teamwork and collaboration

Many games require players to play in pairs, teams and collaborate with others for the greatest outcome. Negotiating what tools to use, trusting others to have your back in battle and deciding on the best course of action as a team can all be great ways to learn those important skills of working with others, compromise and trust that may well transfer to the work they do both at school and beyond.

WHAT SCARES US ABOUT GAMING

There are certainly some elements of gaming that can give us some cause for concern. Here are the key things I believe gaming is something parents feel overwhelmed by:

- **The ease of access.** With mobile devices, the games can now be accessed just about anywhere at any time.

- **The time-wasting.** Because of that ease of access there is an assumption that any time they are playing games then that is time that could really be spent doing something else. And the way in which they hook us in makes this battle with time even more challenging.

- **The content.** Obviously some of the games on the market are completely inappropriate for young people and the themes and detail can be very graphic, very violent and misogynistic. Not something we want young people exposed to, but unfortunately so many are.

- **The violent or aggressive behaviours.** Whilst the research is still inconclusive about whether violent video games lead to violent behaviours, it can be said that some parents find their child becomes more moody or aggressive when they are playing games or as soon as they are told to get off.

While these concerns can feel overwhelming, it's important to remember that they are generally concerns that we can manage, take control of and prevent from taking over with just a few conscious choices around our kids' gaming habits.

HOW TO SPOT A PROBLEM

The creators of games know what appeals to our brain and our reward systems and thus they come complete with hooks and never-ending loop systems that make it very difficult for us to put them down. With the lure of getting to one more level, making one more kill, finding one more bag of loot, crushing one more piece of candy, having one more chance to be the last man standing, the brain of a young person can find it difficult to naturally tell themself when they have had enough. So we do need to help them with that.

That means we can have some boundaries around the times they play, particularly if they are having trouble regulating that for themselves. And we must look out for the red flags that tell us our children are struggling to control their time spent. We want to avoid them heading down the slippery slope to obsessive behaviours that get harder to manage the older they get, and the more entrenched those behaviours become.

Red flags may be:

- having a tantrum or becoming aggressive when they are told to come off the games
- skipping meals or losing sleep because of game playing
- no longer participating in activities they once enjoyed
- slipping in school grades or not wanting to attend school.

The problem, of course, is that all of the above can also be seen as normal tween and teen behaviours. But if we think that our child's game playing is impacting other areas of their life in an increasingly negative way, then it may be time to step in and make some changes. Discuss together those concerns and how you can come up

Games come
complete with hooks
and never-ending
loop systems that
make it very difficult
for us to put them
down.

with a plan to help them remain in control and avoid slipping into those obsessive behaviours.

HOW TO DECIDE WHICH GAMES ARE OKAY

Like the books we read, the media we consume and the foods we eat, there are certainly some video games that are healthier, more helpful and have many benefits that many others may not have. Choosing the right games to play can also determine the extent of the benefit they provide.

Kids being kids will usually gravitate to the popular games their peers are playing and want to hang out in the places where their mates are. Sometimes these places can be appropriate and healthy, and sometimes they can be completely wrong for their stage of development, their understanding and their wellbeing. If your child wants a particular game and you are unsure if they are ready, there are a number of things you can do:

1. Research the game by reading reviews and finding out age recommendations and themes or concepts related to the game that may affect different ages and stages.

2. Watch someone else play. You can easily Google a game and watch other people playing the game on YouTube. After only a few minutes you will usually get a feel for the themes, language,

concepts, level of violence and appropriateness. Certainly enough to help you determine whether it is suitable for your child.

3. Head to sites such as **commonsensemedia.org** who give reviews and recommendations on every game, app, movie and media that is out there.

4. Play the game with your child. If you have decided a game may be okay but there are a few things you may need to discuss, then have a go at playing with your child. You don't have to do it for hours but enough to be able to point out any concerns or have any conversations you may need to have. It also may well become a great way for you to have some fun and bond with your child which has often been reported as a great byproduct.

If you make a decision that your child is not ready for a particular game, you may well get the cries of 'but everybody else is allowed'. And I guess this is part of parenting. We make decisions based on what we think is best for our child based on our own set of values and beliefs. This has been around for eons and it will likely hang around for many more. Our differing belief systems, values, family circumstances and lifestyles all mean that families are going to come to different conclusions about what is and isn't appropriate for their kids.

HELPING THE OBSESSIVE GAMER

Dealing with a child whose gaming is getting out of control can be pretty overwhelming.

The first thing you need them to know is your reasons for wanting to make changes to their gaming are not because you want to spoil all their fun or dictate how they spend their time. Rather, you want to ensure they're maintaining control of their time and the effects the games are having on them. You also don't want these conversations to occur when they are in the middle of a game and emotionally invested in that game.

If you have a child who is bigger than you, has become aggressive and is refusing to heed your requests for compromise, they may have gone past the stage of talking to you about their gaming and slipped into an obsessive pattern of behaviour. It's extremely difficult for them to manage or make any changes when they're in that state. If you feel you've exhausted all possibilities of regaining control, then it's time to seek professional help. There are often other factors at play that need to be dealt with in a professional way.

SIMPLE RULES FOR HAPPY, HEALTHY GAMING

Whenever I stipulate rules for families around gaming or technology, I always stress that it's not my place to tell parents every rule and boundary they should have. I'd rather give parents lots of information and suggest some rules and boundaries that might work.

From there; however, it's really up to you to apply the rules and guidelines that you believe will help your particular situation, your particular challenges and meet your individual child's needs.

Here are some suggestions that may help you manage your child's video game playing:

- Look at your individual child and see how they are coping with their gaming. If they start missing meals, throwing tantrums, missing sports practice and neglecting pets, chores, homework or other people, then you might want to make some changes.

- Discuss with them why you might need to make some changes or have those time limits or boundaries.

- Have discussions about video game playing away from the games. You are unlikely to get a decent response whilst they are in the midst of battle or just about to be the last man standing in Fortnite.

- Play it with them. You might like it. It could be a good way to bond. You might not like it. That's okay too, but showing an interest and finding out about the appeal makes it easier for us to relate and easier to parent them.

- Make use of settings buttons. There are so many ways games can be made safer and can promote a far more positive experience if you go and check out the settings. It may be you can block who can talk to your child, who can request them as a friend, what language they hear, what content they view, who can chat, comment etc.

- Make sure your child also knows how to block and report people.

- Avoid putting gaming consoles in the bedroom. We know the games are hard enough to resist for our young people with underdeveloped brains and capacity to always regulate their timing and behaviour, so why make it so much harder for them by putting a gaming console right under their nose. The last thing they need is to reach for a controller in the middle of the night to play 'just one game'.

- Avoid headphones for younger users so you can hear conversations and be alert to any sharing of private information or bullying behaviours.

- Make it clear to other parents if you have a problem with your child playing a certain game when they go on playdates.

There are so many
ways games can be
made safer and can
promote a far more
positive experience if
you go and check out
the settings.

- Always insist on leaving the game to eat a meal. Preferably with the family at the dinner table but I wouldn't be letting them play games whilst eating meals.

- You can build a real culture of 'balanced play' in your homes. The games are just one of many ways they need to be entertained or hang out with mates. Provide many other opportunities to get out, be active and connect in real life.

- Having another activity for them to go on with once a game is finished, especially something active or even rough and tumble if a more active/ violent game has been played can really help. This helps to reduce the levels of adrenaline and expel the cortisol that has accumulated playing these types of games. Also, skin to skin contact or even a cuddle can help release the oxytocin. Gaming can result in an overloaded sensory system, so giving them an active transition activity can actually help them to calm themselves down.

- Rejoice in some of the positive elements of game playing. Praise their teamwork, perseverance, trial and error or thinking outside the box that has taken place in order for them to get to a new level, build a new fortress or even win the battle.

Like all things in a digital world, gaming can be a positive and beneficial way to spend one's time or it can negatively impact a person's wellbeing. Once again, it is the behaviours, the habits and the types of experiences we are having on the games, that will determine the extent to which they can remain a positive addition to our children's lives.

Things to ponder

- Does my child have control over their time gaming?
- Does their mood change when they stop playing a game?
- Are they still getting enough sleep, eating properly, keeping up with schoolwork, friends and chores?
- Could this be something we occasionally do together?

Conversations to have with your kids

- Do you enjoy positive interactions with others playing games?
- What is it you enjoy about playing video games?
- Are there times when the games are not so enjoyable?
- Does your frustration spill over to other aspects of your life?
- Do you get angry when told to get off a game?
- Can you happily transition between gaming and other activities?
- Do you know how to handle abusive comments from others or any unwanted attention?
- Are there any areas of your life that are suffering because of your game playing? Sleep? School? Seeing friends? Staying active?

CHAPTER 11

....

PARENTING a great kid in a digital world

....

Parenting is challenging and we will all get things wrong from time to time. But if we focus on the positive ways we can influence our kids:

- empowering them with the confidence to make good decisions,
- building their resilience to bounce back when the decisions of themselves or others are not helpful,

then we have a pretty good chance of coming out the other end with a pretty great kid.

Here are some things to have in the back of our minds every day we parent.

AIM TO BE A GOOD ROLE MODEL

As a parent, we can talk and instruct and plead and entice our kids to always do the right thing. But we also have to recognise that kids learn much more from what they see and experience than they do from what we say.

When I talk to students about the time they spend online and the need to have plenty of time for other experiences, or the need to come to the dinner table without a device, I always get at least one child either put up their hand or come to me later and say, 'That thing you said about putting your phones away, well my mum/dad/grandma is the worst. She always has her phone in her hand and is continually doing things on it. She says they are important things but then is the first to tell us off'.

Now I have no way of knowing whether these kids' parents are doing important things on their phone, but I do know we have to be mindful of the messages our actions are sending to our kids.

Additionally, one only has to read the comments section of popular blogs and online news articles to see how heinous adults can be when talking to each other. What do those abusive, vitriolic comments say to their children about appropriate ways to behave online?

Here's how you can be a good role model:

- Look at how you use your phone around other people. Are you putting it down to give someone your full attention or are you continuing to scroll whilst they are trying to talk to you?

- Do you set aside time to answer emails, scroll your social network feeds or post pictures at a time of day that is not interrupting other important moments or events?

- Are you mindful of how you talk to other people online? Even if it's an issue you are passionate about, are you staying on topic and discussing the issues at hand, rather than being judgemental and getting lost in personal attacks on others?

LOOK OUT FOR TEACHABLE MOMENTS

You don't have to look far every day to find teachable moments in the online world:

- There are celebrities losing sponsorship deals because of a racist or sexist tweet.

- There are politicians having past transgressions dug up to reveal a set of ethics that don't align with their current party position.

- There are people losing their jobs for having a whinge via their social media feed about their lazy boss.

Recognise that kids
learn much more
from what they see
and experience than
they do from what
we say.

- There are people whose indiscretions are caught on video or tracking devices that don't put them in the place they were meant to be.
- There are the kids having their group chat that have forgotten their mates' parents do spot checks and are now privy to the nasty conversations that may be taking place.

We don't want to make our kids so afraid that every single thing they do is going to come back to haunt them in some way. But we do want them to remember that negative online behaviours are there for all to see and can have repercussions for them. In pointing out those moments where others have not been so aware of their digital footprint, we are able to continue to alert them to the ways this world can work, and the need for us to continue to aim for control over how the rest of the world sees us.

When we do so, we want to do it in a way that offers conversation and discusses other alternatives or ways people could have handled situations differently. Remember, when we lecture our kids constantly, or we sit them down to hear a lesson on what not to do online, we can tend to get the eye roll and the glazed look that usually translates to tuning out. So bring it up as conversation and turn the focus from what 'not to do' into 'what could we do' instead.

RECONSIDER TAKING AWAY SCREENS AS PUNISHMENT

Many people find that taking the devices away from kids when they do the wrong thing is the one sure-fire way to make it clear to them that behaviour won't be tolerated. While this can certainly be a somewhat effective way of letting a younger child know there are consequences for their actions, we have to be really careful about using devices as punishment as they get older.

As the screens become increasingly embedded in their lives, they rely on them for a lot of their social connection and even their downtime and entertainment. If we threaten to take them away at the first sign of trouble, we risk them shutting down and not coming to us if they find themselves in situations that may be getting out of hand. And we don't want that. We want them to be able to learn from that mistake, find out ways to make it better and look for other ways to reinforce better behaviours. It doesn't mean we can't reduce the amount of time they have access, or take access away at certain times of the day or night. But we do not want to contribute to the 'us versus them' scenario, and further alienate them from our ability to guide and support.

ALLOW YOUR CHILD TO MAKE MISTAKES

Remember that while this stuff all feels relatively new to you, it is even more so for our kids. Despite their seemingly innate knowledge of technology and devices, learning to live, connect, interact, manage emotions, prioritise their time and maintain control of their worlds, is still very much in the learning phases regardless of their ages. We have to understand and accept that they will make mistakes.

- They will say the wrong thing at times.
- They may overshare.
- They may forget about all the different beliefs or circumstances of their large group of followers.
- They may let time slip away as they indulge in 12 too many YouTube videos or games of Fortnite.
- They may accidentally post a video that has questionable song lyrics.
- They may get wrapped up in a disagreement with someone that is unlikely to be resolved in any polite manner.

When they make those mistakes, we want them to feel they have the skills to rectify, or apologise, or to try and make it right. And if we make ourselves available to help with those mistakes, rather than have them scared to acknowledge them, then the mistakes they make will continue to be small ones they can learn from, and not the catastrophic ones that can change their lives.

CREATE STRONG RITUALS AND ROUTINES FOR SAFETY AND SECURITY

Studies have shown that when kids feel secure, and when they feel heard, they are far more likely to show characteristics of resilience which we know is something that many need in abundance today.

A great way to provide both of those things is at the family mealtime. Of course, circumstances don't always allow for us to sit down every night at the same time with all members of the family home to enjoy this time. But we can certainly find enough mealtimes a week to make this happen, free of devices. This gives kids space and time to be heard and to connect. I know for my own boys, when they get home from school the last thing they want to do is sit and have long discussions about their day. They need some downtime to process the day's events, to chill out and have some time without questions. But come time for dinner, they are ready to chat, argue, interrupt each other and share their good and bad.

And it's not just mealtime routines that give kids this security. It can be a bedtime story. It can be Saturday morning milkshakes after basketball. It can be annual weekends away or camping trips. It can be Friday night board games, movie nights or summertime backyard cricket. There doesn't even need to be a lot of talking. It's the reliability and comfort that comes with these ritualistic experiences that can be crucial to a child's sense of belonging.

We also know that this sense of belonging helps give kids the confidence to enjoy positive relationships outside the family home, both online and in real life. In a world where resilience is going to be an essential element of living and interacting in a positive manner, we need to take every opportunity we can to help provide kids with the stable, supportive environments that help them build on that resilience, and nurture their sense of self-confidence and place in the world.

ESTABLISH STRONG FAMILY VALUES AND RULES

Families today are vastly different in their experiences, their circumstances, their backgrounds, their environments and their daily living. What is super important to one family, may not be so important to

A sense of belonging
helps give kids the
confidence to enjoy
positive relationships
outside the
family home.

another, and thus they make their rules and boundaries based around those things that are important to them. That is why some families will go to church every week and others won't. Some families have a low sugar diet and don't have sweets or lollies in the house. Some families allow their children to stay up until 8.30 pm. Some allow the kids to decide when their bedtime is, and others stick to a 7 pm bedtime routine.

You now have a lot of knowledge about what is out there when it comes to the digital world and the challenges faced by us all. So with that knowledge and your beliefs and values about how you want your life and the lives of your children to play out, go ahead and make the rules and boundaries that will help serve that purpose.

- If that means no phones should be in the bedroom because you are passionate about giving kids downtime and lots of sleep, then make that a rule.

- If you are concerned that obsessive behaviours about devices take your child away from their studies, then make a rule to prevent that happening.

- If connecting on a nightly basis at the dinner table is something you see as a no-brainer then you will probably want to make a non-negotiable rule of no devices at the dinner table.

We are never going to all have the same rules and play out our lives in the same manner. And that's okay. Just make sure you are doing what you can to achieve what you want as a way of life for your family. There really are lots of ways to raise a great kid.

····························
Things to ponder
····························

- How do I frame my own conversations about the digital world with my kids?
- Could I adopt a more positive mindset to help them feel comfortable in coming to me should things go wrong?
- What would my kids think I would do, should I find out they did something wrong online?

Conversations to have with your kids

- Would you feel comfortable coming to me if you made a mistake online?

- Do you have other people you would turn to should you find yourself in trouble?

- How do you think our values are reflected in some of the rules we have around technology?

- Do you think the rules and boundaries we have are fair?

- What are some of your favourite rituals we do as a family? Can you think of any others you would like to incorporate?

- Do you think I, as a parent, set a good example using technology and screens?

- What ways do you think I could improve and be a better role model?

CONCLUSION

As I mentioned in the introduction of this book, it can be overwhelming trying to keep up with the ever-changing landscape of the online world. As fast as we get our heads around one social media app, another one becomes 'all the rage'. Just when we feel like we understand the game our child gets huge enjoyment out of, suddenly they're playing a completely new one with all their friends.

My hope is this book gives you the confidence of knowing that all the things you're doing to be a good parent in the 'real' world also helps you be a good parent of kids who spend a lot of time interacting online.

Continue to refer back to this book for the 'macro' strategies around parenting a kid in the digital age. Meanwhile, if you're looking for the 'micro' stuff—a breakdown of the latest apps and the latest ways kids are using technology to interact, head to my blog: **themodernparent.net**.

That's where I can:

- give you strategies to help you deal with techno tantrums
- keep you updated on the red flags that indicate your child may not be coping
- give you ideas on how to make rules that allow for better functioning of your tech lives
- alert you to ways of being more mindful about your families use of technology
- give you strategies to avoid the pervasiveness of digital distraction
- recommend software, systems and settings to help you protect your child from the pornographic and inappropriate content that constantly threatens to seep into their screens.

I want to continue to empower you to:

- have informed conversations with your kids
- be able to talk frankly about the challenges rather than just lecturing about the risks
- nurture and explore the positive experiences, people and pursuits to follow online
- listen to your kids.=

- make boundaries for your family that will work for your circumstances
- help your kid make boundaries for themselves
- help them develop healthy self-esteem that transcends all the comparison and exclusion and petty comments that pervade their social feeds
- continue to instil values of kindness and empathy
- create that culture of balance.

And remember to focus on the most important connection of all, the one you have with your child.

If we give all of the above a pretty good shot, my anecdotal evidence, and increasingly the scientific evidence, continue to show me that we will more than likely end up with really great kids who have the confidence and resilience to operate happily and healthily in an increasingly digital world.

ACKNOWLEDGEMENTS

A big thank you must firstly go to my editor Kelly Exeter. Kelly and I have known each other for some time and, while being mentored by her at a business mastermind run by Darren Rowse and the ProBlogger team, she encouraged me to write this book. Her skill at putting all my words and thoughts and rambles into something that is clear and concise and easy to consume is something I'm so thankful for. She also beautifully designed the cover of the book as well as the interior. A woman of many talents!

I would also like to thank my friend Darren Rowse, not only for all that I learnt on that mastermind, but for encouraging me to start a blog nearly 10 years ago. That blog led me to build a business that I'm hugely passionate about and has allowed me to connect with so many amazing people, visit so many schools, travel the country, engage with fabulous teachers and learn from many wonderful students.

I would also like to thank Michael Grose who both wrote the foreword to this book and told me, 'You definitely have a book in you. I really think you should write one.' It was pretty amazing for me to hear those words from Michael since I have been a huge fan of his work and his common sense approach to parenting from the moment I had my first son 20 years ago. His words combined with Kelly's encouragement left me no choice really!

Thank you to my wonderful mum and dad for your love and support, for instilling in me the importance of family and for providing me with the greatest of parenting role models.

To all of my beautiful family and friends for their ongoing support and encouragement and of course to my amazing husband Paul, a fabulous father to our kids and always there to sing my praises and encourage every step of the way.

And last but definitely not least, my darling baby girl for being the inspiration for everything that I do and of course my beautiful boys, who really are great kids.

www.ingramcontent.com/pod-product-compliance
Lightning Source LLC
Chambersburg PA
CBHW060039030426
42334CB00019B/2403